María del Pilar Díaz Martínez

Evaluation and diagnosis of trigger points in physiotherapy

María del Pilar Díaz Martínez

Evaluation and diagnosis of trigger points in physiotherapy

Part One: Upper limb

ScienciaScripts

Imprint
Any brand names and product names mentioned in this book are subject to trademark, brand or patent protection and are trademarks or registered trademarks of their respective holders. The use of brand names, product names, common names, trade names, product descriptions etc. even without a particular marking in this work is in no way to be construed to mean that such names may be regarded as unrestricted in respect of trademark and brand protection legislation and could thus be used by anyone.

Cover image: www.ingimage.com

This book is a translation from the original published under ISBN 978-613-9-44172-3.

Publisher:
Sciencia Scripts
is a trademark of
Dodo Books Indian Ocean Ltd. and OmniScriptum S.R.L publishing group

120 High Road, East Finchley, London, N2 9ED, United Kingdom
Str. Armeneasca 28/1, office 1, Chisinau MD-2012, Republic of Moldova, Europe
Printed at: see last page
ISBN: 978-620-3-55941-5

Index

1. INTRODUCTION TO PHYSIOTHERAPY AND MYOFASCIAL TRIGGER POINTS (MGP).

1.1. History and development of physical therapy.

The history of physical therapy dates back to ancient times, where physical agents such as water, heat and massage were used in combination with magical or religious rituals to cure illnesses. In ancient Greece, Hippocrates promoted self-healing of the body by natural means and mentioned the therapeutic use of water and massage. During the Middle Ages, there was a decline in the use of these methods due to religious prohibitions, but in the Renaissance, the classical approach was resumed and massage therapy was recommended for various ailments. In the 16th and 17th centuries, works were published highlighting the importance of physical exercise and massotherapy for health. In the 18th century, authors such as Antonio Perez Escobar and Joseph Clement Tissot advocated the incorporation of physical exercise in medical treatment. In the 19th century, with the advent of evolutionism and positivism, there were great advances in medicine and science, although physical agents still did not occupy a prominent place compared to surgery and pharmacology. During this period, important contributions were made in the field of physiotherapy, such as the development of physical education by Pehr Henrik Ling, the introduction of mechanotherapy by Zander, and the studies of electrostimulation by Duchenne De Boulogne. These advances laid the foundation for the evolution of physiotherapy as a therapeutic discipline in the following centuries (1).

During the 20th century, physiotherapy underwent a significant development that marked its consolidation as a health care discipline. In the early years of the century, the publication of the "Library of therapeutics of Gilbert and Carnot" introduced the term "physiotherapy" and classified physical agents for the first time. Prominent practitioners such as Frenkel, Klapp and Lovett, among others, made important contributions to the treatment of various conditions, from cerebellar disorders to scoliosis and muscular imbalances. In 1933, Guthrie-Smith developed the apparatus that would bear his name, which laid the foundation for what is known today as poleotherapy. In 1946, Delorme and Watkins designed a systematic muscle strengthening method called "progressive resistance exercises", contributing to the evolution in the treatment of muscle strength. Françoise Mézières initiated the study of muscle chains in 1949, laying the foundations of modern techniques such as global postural reeducation and the muscle chain technique. Herman Kabat developed the proprioceptive neuromuscular facilitation method in the 1940s, focusing on muscular potentiation and proprioception. In 1958, the World Health Organization (WHO) defined physiotherapy as "the art and science of treatment by means of therapeutic exercise, heat, cold, water, massage and electricity". In 1967, the World Confederation for Physical Therapy (WCPT) described it as "the art and science of physical treatment," focusing on the use of physical agents to cure, prevent, recover and readapt patients. The Bobath couple introduced a treatment technique for infantile cerebral palsy, which was later extended to the treatment of adults with hemiplegia. In 1967, Hislop and Perrine developed the concept of "isokinetic work", which revolutionized treatment by means of resistance proportional to the muscular force exerted. Václav Vojta published in 1974 a system of early diagnosis and treatment based on postural reactivity, especially relevant in the pediatric field (2).

Among the events of physiotherapy in Spain, March 2, 1969 stands out, with a meeting in Madrid that marked the beginning of the foundation of the Spanish Association of Physiotherapists (AEF). Subsequently, on June 12, 1969, in Barcelona, the Constituent Assembly was held where the first National Board of Directors, led by José Llopis Diez, was approved and confirmed. In 1970, the AEF underwent significant changes with the election of a new board of directors during an assembly in Alicante, headed by Mr. Roberto González Fernández. That same year, the AEF joined the European Confederation of Physiotherapists, strengthening its position at the international level. The AEF was dedicated to promoting the elevation of physiotherapy studies to university level, working closely with the Ministry of Education to establish the University Schools of Physiotherapy in line with international standards. During the following years, the AEF worked on the elaboration of a new curriculum for physiotherapy, leading a national commission in charge of this project. In 1972, the association submitted to the Ministry of Education a project for the restructuring of physiotherapy studies, which eventually led to the promulgation of a Royal Decree in 1980, establishing the basis for the creation of the University Schools of Physiotherapy. In parallel, the AEF consolidated its international presence by being recognized as a full member of the World Confederation of Physiotherapists in 1974. In addition, it continued to promote the profession nationally, organizing events and conferences, and launching the magazine "Fisioterapia" in 1979. In June of that year, a general assembly was held in which a new national board of directors was elected, led by Mr. Roberto Núñez Pérez, marking the beginning of a new era for physiotherapy in Spain (3).

Physiotherapy experienced significant progress in Spain from the 1980s onwards, with important milestones that contributed to its development and recognition as a university degree and health profession. In 1980, physiotherapy was established as a university degree in Spain, but it was in 1987, with the University Reform Law, when it received an important boost. During these years, the Spanish Association of Physiotherapists (AEF) made active efforts in favor of the growth of the profession. In 1985, the AEF adapted its Statutes to the new territorial organization, and in 1989, the Official University Degree in Physiotherapy was officially established. The integration of the physiotherapist in the Primary Care team, promoted by the AEF, marked an important milestone in 1989, followed by a more detailed regulation in 1991. In addition, in 1989, the "Specific Area of Knowledge of Physiotherapy" was consolidated, allowing physiotherapists access to academic positions (3).

In 1990, the I International Congress of Sports Physiotherapy in Spain was held in Valladolid. However, the most significant milestone was the foundation of the first professional association of physiotherapists in the country: the Association of Physiotherapists of Catalonia, supported and financed by the Spanish Association of Physiotherapists (AEF). This step marked the beginning of the creation of professional associations in all the autonomous communities, making the members of the AEF the first members of the association. In 1998, the General Council of Colleges of Physiotherapists of Spain defined physiotherapy as "the science and art of physical treatment", focused on the use of physical means to cure, prevent disease and promote health. In 1999, the World Confederation for Physical Therapy (WCPT) updated the definition of physical therapy, emphasizing that it is a service provided by physical therapists, which includes assessment, diagnosis, planning, intervention and evaluation, and that complete and functional movement is fundamental to health. In 2001, the AEF commemorated the 50th anniversary of the WCPT and signed an agreement to organize its XIV World Congress. Scientific publications were also promoted. In 2002, Mrs. Antonia Gómez Conesa became the first physiotherapist to obtain a University Chair. These events marked significant milestones in the consolidation and recognition of physiotherapy as a vital health profession in Spain (4).

Throughout the following years, significant milestones have been reached in the development and promotion of physiotherapy in Spain. In 2003, the XIV WCPT Congress was held in Barcelona and the Permanent Board of the AEF was renewed. In 2004, the White Paper on the Degree in Physiotherapy was published and the Official College of Physiotherapists of La Rioja was created. Student movements in 2005 advocated for quality training, while in 2006 the Technical Sheet for Undergraduate Studies in Physiotherapy was published and the foundations were laid for the Iberoamerican Association of Physiotherapy and Kinesiology. In 2007, the 50th anniversary of physiotherapy in Spain was celebrated and the conditions of the Study Plans for the Degree in Physiotherapy were approved. In 2008, the Permanent Board of the AEF was renewed and the sponsorship of the PEDro database was approved. Since 2012, the Revista Iberoamericana de Fisioterapia y Kinesiología merged with the journal Fisioterapia. In 2012, Madrid hosted the XIV National Congress of Physiotherapy, standing out for its innovation and active participation. In November of that year, during the X Anniversary of the Professional Association of Physiotherapists of Extremadura, Ms. Antonia Gómez Conesa was elected as president of the Permanent Board. In December 2014, new regulations were approved to improve the functioning of the AEF and it was decided that Antonia Gómez would continue as editor of the journal after her presidency. During this decade, the AEF promoted the creation of specialized affiliate associations, such as the Spanish Association of Physiotherapists in Mental Health and others. She collaborated with the ER-WCPT in the creation of the European Physiotherapy Guidelines for Parkinson's Disease. From 2010 to 2016, Sonia Souto represented the AEF as Second Vice Chairman of the ER-WCPT. The AEF actively participated with the Ministry of Health in various strategies and projects, such as the IMA Project (Intelligent Motion Analysis) and the Commitment to Quality of Scientific Societies Project. In 2016, the journal Fisioterapia obtained the seal of Quality of Scientific Journals. In addition, the AEF organized two international events in Madrid in collaboration with WCPT (1).

According to Royal Decree 1001/2002 of September 27, 2002, physiotherapy is a health profession that focuses on the prevention, evaluation, diagnosis and treatment of musculoskeletal and neurological disorders, as well as on promoting the well-being and quality of life of the individual. It is based on the use of manual techniques, therapeutic exercises, physical agents and patient education to restore physical function and improve mobility, strength and flexibility. Physiotherapy addresses both acute and chronic dysfunctions, working in collaboration with other health professionals to achieve the best results for the patient (5).

The function is what defines the exercise of a profession. According to the statute of the General Council of Colleges of Physiotherapists, Chapter I of the basic principles of the practice of Physiotherapy, in Article 1 Of Physiotherapy we find that Physiotherapy is the study and art of physical treatment, that is, the set of methods, actions and techniques that, through the application of physical means, heal and prevent disease, promote health, recover, train, rehabilitate and readapt people affected by psychophysical dysfunctions or those who want to maintain an adequate level of health. The practice of Physiotherapy also includes the performance by the physiotherapist, alone or in a multidisciplinary team, of electrical and manual tests aimed at determining the degree of affectation of innervation and muscle strength, tests to determine functional capacities, range of joint movement and measures of vital capacity, all focused on determining the physiotherapeutic evaluation and diagnosis, as a preliminary step to any act of physiotherapy, as well as the use of diagnostic aids to monitor the evolution of users. The ultimate goal of physiotherapy is to promote, maintain, restore and increase the level of health of citizens in order to improve the quality of life of the person and facilitate their full social reintegration (5).

In Article 2 of the Physiotherapists, we find the responsibilities of the physiotherapist, whether in terms of care, teaching, research or management, derive directly from the primary role of physiotherapy in society. These responsibilities are carried out in accordance with the fundamental ethical principles that govern all professional practice. This implies a profound respect for the dignity of the person, the protection of their human rights, as well as a marked responsibility, honesty and sincerity in all interactions with users. Within these responsibilities is the task of establishing and applying a wide range of physical means with therapeutic effects in treatments for users of various medical and surgical specialties. These physical means include, among others, the application of electricity, heat, cold, massage, water, air, movement, light and specialized therapeutic exercises. Such interventions are applied in areas such as cardiopulmonary, orthopedics, neurological injuries, pre- and postpartum maternity, among others. It also includes the performance of specific manual procedures and treatments, alternative or complementary, within the field of physiotherapy (5).

These responsibilities are performed in a variety of settings, ranging from health institutions to educational centers, sports facilities, physical therapy offices, rehabilitation centers and gyms, among others. Once physical therapists comply with the requirements established by the applicable legislation, they acquire full rights and faculties to practice their profession, regardless of the modality or legal title under which they provide their services. It is important to emphasize that the free practice of the profession of physical therapist takes place in a context of free competition and is subject to specific regulations, particularly with regard to the offer of services and the determination of remuneration, in accordance with current legislation on antitrust and unfair competition (5).

1.2. History of myofascial trigger points (MTrPs).

The understanding of musculoskeletal pain has advanced significantly, focusing on identifying specific sources and causes, such as neuropathic, joint dysfunction, muscular causes and pain modulation by the central nervous system. The history of muscle pain was extensively reviewed during the 20th century and recently updated, highlighting the publications that underpin our current understanding of trigger point (TP) myofascial pain.

In the 19th century, Froriep described "Muskel Sch wiele" as palpable and painful hardnesses in the muscles, while Adler in America used the term "muscular rheumatism" and introduced the concept of pain radiating from tender points. In England, Gowers, Stockman and Llewellyn Jones introduced the term "fibrositis", while in Germany, Schmidt used "Muskelrheumatismus". Schade, in 1919, discovered that muscle stiffness persisted even after death, suggesting that the cause was not active muscle contraction, and proposed the term "Myogelosen". During the following decades, several researchers, such as F. Lange and M. Lange, contributed to the understanding of muscle responses and PGs. In 1937, Hans Kraus first used ethyl chloride spray to treat "Muskelhiirten" and subsequently PGs. Kellgren, in 1938, demonstrated referred pain patterns by injecting saline into muscles. In this same period, three physicians, Michael Gutstein, Michael Kelly and Janet Travell, identified myofascial PGs in different regions of the world, each using different diagnostic terms, but describing similar characteristics such as palpable hardness, points of extreme tenderness, referred pain and relief by massage or infiltration. Travell, in particular, had a lasting influence with over 40 articles published between 1942 and 1990, and his "Manual of Trigger Points" published in 1983 and 1992, where he documented PG pain patterns in 32 skeletal muscles (6).

Pathologic studies have attempted to identify the cause of PGs. Miehlke and colleagues conducted an extensive study on fibrositis, finding dystrophic findings in more symptomatic cases. The relationship between fibromyalgia and PGs has been a matter of debate, but in 1990, a group of rheumatologists established diagnostic criteria for fibromyalgia, linking it to central nervous system dysfunction. In the mid-1980s, A. Fischer developed a pressure algometer to measure PG sensitivity and hypersensitive points in fibromyalgia (6).

Finally, recent needle EMG studies by Hubbard and Berkoff in 1993 and rabbit experiments by Hong and Torigoe in 1994 confirmed that a dysfunctional motor plate area is the main location of PG pathophysiology. An additional advance was the interexaminer reliability study by Gerwin in 1994, which demonstrated reliable identification of myofascial PG criteria in five muscles (6).

1.3. Definition of PGM.

Myofascial pain syndrome (MPS) is a condition characterized by a set of sensory, motor and autonomic signs and symptoms resulting from the presence of myofascial trigger points (MTrPs). These MTrPs are hyperirritable areas within a tight band of skeletal muscle, which present as palpable nodules and are painful when pressed, stretched or contracted (6). In addition to localized pain, PGMs can cause referred pain, motor dysfunction, and autonomic phenomena, such as changes in skin temperature or abnormal sweating and have a diameter between 2 and 5 mm. To diagnose MDS, it is crucial to identify all PGMs that contribute to symptoms, even if some of them are not clinically active. MDS can affect a single muscle (monomuscular MDS) or involve muscle groups or broader anatomical regions (7).

The concept of MTrPs has evolved since the term was introduced by orthopedic surgeon A. Steindler in 1940, who observed that novocaine infiltrations into these points relieved certain muscle pain. However, the most commonly used definition for trigger points is that provided by Janet Travell and David Simons in 1992 "A myofascial trigger point (MTrP) is a muscle point that is extremely irritable, associated with a palpable hypersensitive nodule within a tight band". They were among the pioneers in researching and publishing on MTrPs, developing a manual that has become a reference for subsequent studies. Historically, PGMs have been known by various names, which has led to confusion. However, the terminology developed by Travell and Simons has been widely accepted in the scientific community. These trigger points, when found in skeletal muscles, can trigger referred pain, hypersensitivity and dysfunction, making accurate diagnosis and appropriate treatment essential (8).

1.4. Importance of PGMs in Physical Therapy

The skeletal musculature, the largest organ of the human body and accounting for almost 50% of body weight, is made up of approximately 400 muscles. These muscles can develop myofascial trigger points (TTPs) that cause pain and motor dysfunction, sometimes radiating to other areas. It cannot be stated that all painful points to the touch are MTPs, to consider it a trigger point we must observe other characteristics that will be detailed later in the section on trigger point diagnosis. This type of pain complicates diagnosis and can lead to inadequate treatment. At least 30% of the population experiences muscular symptoms, and many cases correspond to myofascial syndrome (MFS), a common but underdiagnosed problem, especially because it does not always present visible alterations in imaging tests or analysis (9).

MFS is a disabling condition, especially in the working age population, and although it is treatable, its effective management requires not only pain relief, but also correction of structural and postural problems. Correct diagnosis and treatment of this condition is crucial to improve the quality of life of patients (10). MPS is related to various musculoskeletal complaints such as low back pain (11), cervical pain (12), headaches (13, 14) or scapular pain (15). MMPs can be either the primary cause of pain or a secondary complication of other pathologies. Although myofascial pain is not life-threatening, it can severely affect quality of life.

It is essential to differentiate MFS from other disorders, such as fibromyalgia, because although they share certain symptoms, their treatments are different. Fibromyalgia, which is a different condition from MDS, has been linked to MDS because of the similarity in some of its symptoms. Fibromyalgia is characterized by a central sensitization process that causes widespread pain in various tissues, including muscles. In order to advance fibromyalgia research and to facilitate its diagnosis and classification, 18 specific pressure pain points have been identified, most of which overlap with myofascial trigger points. This overlap, together with the lack of knowledge of MDS and the difficulties in diagnosing it, has led to confusion and misdiagnosis. It is very common for people with fibromyalgia to also have MDS, but it does not occur with the same frequency in the reverse direction (16).

The cost associated with myofascial pain is high and mostly avoidable. Many people suffer persistent pain that could improve with proper diagnosis and treatment. Failure to recognize the myofascial nature of pain leads to misdiagnosis, creating frustration and hindering effective treatment. It is crucial that healthcare professionals improve their training and understanding of myofascial PGs to reduce the suffering and costs associated with untreated chronic pain. In addition, increasing research and outreach about this condition can optimize treatments and improve patients' quality of life (16).

1.5. Epidemiology of PGMs.

Myofascial trigger points (TP) are extremely common and affect a large percentage of the population. In a study of 200 asymptomatic young adults, 54% of women and 45% of men were found to have PGs in the muscles of the shoulder girdle. In addition, 25% of these subjects with latent PGs experienced referred pain. In another study of 269 nursing students, PGs were identified in 54% of the right lateral pterygoid muscles, 45% of the right deep right masseter muscles, 43% of the anterior part of the right temporalis muscles, and 40% of the right medial pterygoid muscles. As for the neck muscles, 35% of the head splenius and 33% of the right trapezius showed PG. A neurologist examined 96 patients in a pain clinic and found that in 93% of cases, at least part of the pain was caused by myofascial PGs, being the primary cause of pain in 74% of these patients. Furthermore, in an orthopedic clinic, 21% of patients with musculoskeletal pain had active PGs in the pyramidal muscle (17).

Data show that myofascial PGs are a significant source of pain and dysfunction, with prevalence varying among different studies and populations. However, these trigger points remain underdiagnosed due to a lack of clear diagnostic criteria and insufficient training in this field. This contributes to incorrect diagnoses and unnecessary suffering for patients, in addition to high economic costs due to lost productivity and inadequate treatments. In summary, myofascial PGs affect a significant percentage of the population and are one of the leading causes of musculoskeletal pain, underscoring the need for a greater focus on their diagnosis and proper treatment in clinical practice (17).

2. ANATOMY AND PHYSIOLOGY OF THE PGM.

2.1. PGM physiology.

2.1.1. Muscle structure and function.

Skeletal muscle is composed of fascicles, each containing approximately 100 muscle fibers. Each muscle fiber contains between 1,000 and 2,000 myofibrils, which are chains of sarcomeres connected in series. The sarcomere, the basic contractile unit, consists of actin and myosin filaments that interact to generate contractile force. During contraction, myosin heads, which act as ATPases, bind to actin, driven by ATP energy and activated by calcium released from the sarcoplasmic reticulum. The contractile force of a sarcomere depends on its length; this decreases if the sarcomere is stretched or shortened too much (18).

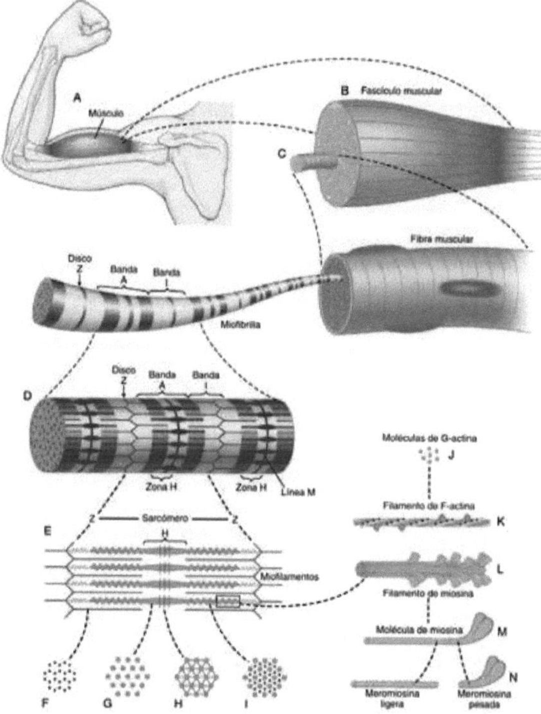

Figure 1. Diagram of the structure and organization of skeletal muscle (18).

2.1.2. Motor unit

The anatomical and functional structure in charge of muscle contraction is called motor unit. This unit is composed of a motor neuron and all the muscle fibers that are controlled by it. The stimulation of a motor neuron causes the activation of all the fibers it innervates; that is, when a motor unit is activated, all its muscle fibers contract. The analysis of the anatomy and physiology of the motor unit has important implications for the diagnosis and monitoring of neuromuscular disorders. The recording of muscle electrical potentials by electrophysiological techniques, such as electromyography (EMG), allows deductions to be made about the muscle structure, its state and function, playing a crucial role in the diagnosis of neuromuscular diseases (19).

The motor unit is the final pathway that allows the central nervous system to control voluntary muscle activity. It is composed of a motor neuron, its axon and all the muscle fibers it innervates. Each muscle fiber is innervated by a single motor neuron, and the motor neuron defines the type of muscle fiber. In postural and limb muscles, a motor unit may comprise between 300 and 1,500 fibers. The propagation of the action potential from the motor neuron to the muscle fibers generates an almost simultaneous contraction of all innervated fibers, resulting in a motor unit action potential. The size of a motor unit and its distribution vary from muscle to muscle, affecting motor control and precision of movements (19).

2.1.3. Motor plates

The motor plate is the structure that connects the motor neuron nerve fiber terminal to the muscle fiber, where the electrical nerve signal is converted into a chemical messenger (acetylcholine) that triggers an electrical signal in the muscle fiber membrane. The region where these motor plates innervate the muscle fibers is known as the "motor point," which is key to the diagnosis and treatment of myofascial trigger points (TP). Motor plaques are usually located near the center of muscle fibers in most skeletal muscles, as shown in studies by Coers and Woolf, and Aquilonius in different human muscles (20).

Understanding the location of the motor plates is crucial for diagnosing and treating PGs. In general, the motor plates are located in the center of the muscle fibers. However, there are exceptions; some muscles, such as rectus abdominis and semitendinosus, have intersections that divide the muscle into segments, each with its own area of motor plates. The sartorius muscle has motor plates scattered throughout the muscle, without a defined zone. This pattern can also be observed in the gracilis muscle, although with variability between individuals. In certain compartmentalized muscles, each compartment has its own zone of motor plates, innervated by a specific branch of the motor nerve, as occurs in the extensor carpi radialis longus and masseter. The gastrocnemius has an angled fiber arrangement that allows for greater strength with less mobility, with the motor plates located along the center of each muscle compartment. The motor plates are aligned transversely to the muscle fibers, following the small neurovascular bundles that cross them. These bundles include sensory and autonomic nerves, whose proximity to the motor plates is relevant to understanding pain and autonomic phenomena associated with PGs (20).

2.1.4. Neuromuscular Junction

In humans, the organization is different from that in animals, cholinesterase staining reveals multiple clusters of synaptic clefts in a motor plate, which could function as several small synapses, explaining the series of spikes in muscle fibers. The neuromuscular junction is a synapse dependent on acetylcholine (ACh) as a neurotransmitter. The nerve terminal releases ACh packets, a process that requires energy produced by mitochondria. When an action potential arrives at the motor neuron, voltage-dependent calcium channels open, allowing the entry of calcium ions that stimulate the release of ACh. ACh is released into the synaptic cleft and crosses to receptors on the postsynaptic membrane of the muscle fiber. Cholinesterase rapidly cleaves ACh, limiting its action and allowing a rapid response to new action potentials. The release of individual ACh packets produces miniature plate potentials, whereas the massive release during an action potential depolarizes the postsynaptic membrane, generating an action potential that propagates along the muscle fiber (20).

In electromyography of active myofascial trigger points, plaque noise is detected, an abnormality that is not observed with the same frequency in healthy muscles. This phenomenon, linked to an abnormal release of acetylcholine at rest in the motor plate of these points, is considered a primary dysfunction in myofascial pain syndrome according to Simons' theory. Studies in animal models have supported this theory, showing that infiltration of botulinum toxin into trigger points reduces plaque noise. Excess acetylcholine causes small bursts of action potentials, resulting in a constant depolarization of the muscle fiber, which generates a sustained shortening known as a contraction knot. This process damages the muscle fiber, creating a cycle of wear and tear that releases nociceptive substances, perpetuating pain and the formation of new trigger points. Myofascial trigger points are also associated with the convergence of painful neural networks in the dorsal root ganglion, which may explain their relationship with various conditions, such as tension headache. Referred pain and hyperalgesia are distinctive features of these points. Rapid local contraction to mechanical stimuli, known as local contractile response, is another feature of myofascial pain syndrome. This response is observed only in muscles with intact innervation and is significantly reduced if the spinal cord connection is interrupted. Chronic pain amplifies nociceptive stimuli, sensitizing spinal cord neurons and facilitating pain transmission. The release of nociceptive substances, such as cytokines and neuropeptides, causes vasodilation and ischemia, contributing to the muscle pain associated with the syndrome (21).

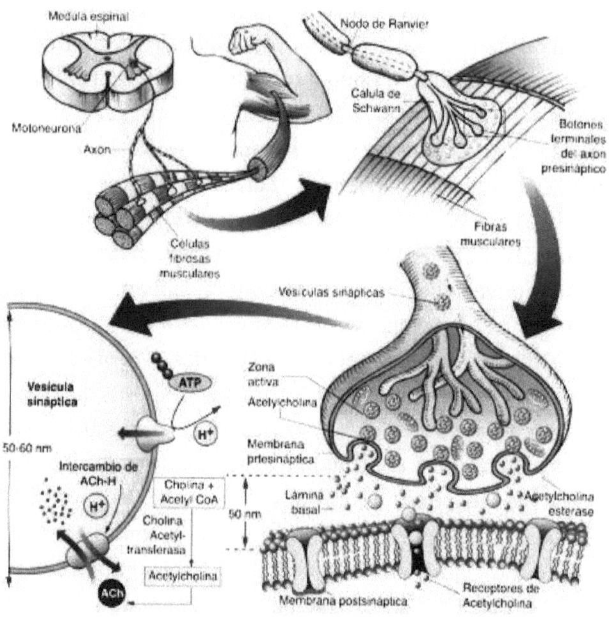

Figure 2. Diagram of the neuromuscular junction: synthesis and release of acetylcholine (22).

2.1.5. Pathophysiology: Biochemical mechanisms of PGMs.

The motor and sensory abnormalities of myofascial trigger points (MTrPs) are not completely understood. MTrPs are thought to result from dysfunctions in the neuromuscular junction and surrounding connective tissue. Electromyographic studies show spontaneous electrical activity (SEA) in MTrPs, possibly caused by excessive release of acetylcholine (ACh), which generates muscle contracture and high metabolic demand. This could explain the presence of tight muscle bands. The "Integrated Trigger Point Hypothesis" suggests that sustained sarcomere contracture and reduced local blood flow cause an energy crisis that perpetuates pain. On the other hand, the "Cinderella Hypothesis" proposes that small muscle fibers, activated during prolonged exertion, become overloaded and contribute to the development of MTrPs. MTrPs are associated with the activation of nociceptors, pain receptors in muscles and surrounding tissues. Various chemical stimuli released during tissue damage (such as bradykinin, serotonin and ATP) contribute to pain and inflammation, and the persistent release of these substances sensitizes nociceptors, increasing pain perception. Peripheral and central sensitization is key in the transition from normal to chronic pain. Peripheral sensitization occurs at the site of injury, while central sensitization occurs when prolonged input of painful signals induces changes in the central nervous system, causing hyperalgesia and allodynia (23).

In myofascial pain syndrome (MPS), active MTrPs can induce changes in spinal cord neurons, expanding areas of pain and causing exaggerated pain responses. Neurotransmitters such as glutamate and substance P (SP) cause neuronal hyperexcitability and long-lasting alterations in the nervous system. Glial cells also release inflammatory cytokines that increase neuronal sensitivity. Microdialysis studies have shown that active MTrPs have elevated levels of substances associated with pain and inflammation compared to normal muscles. Techniques such as dry needling can reduce these substances, relieving pain and stiffness (23).

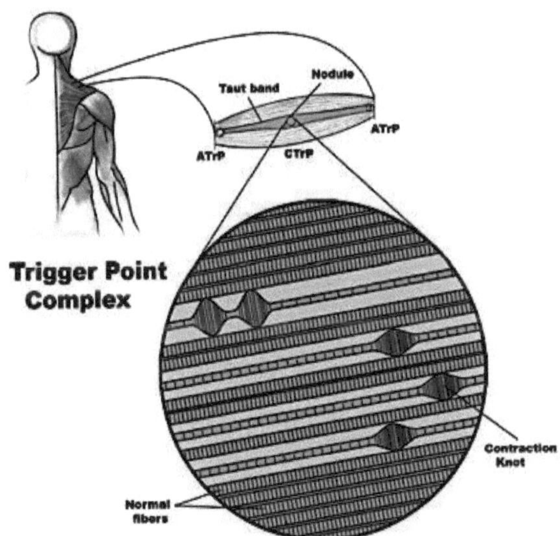

Diagram of a trigger point complex (23).

Roles of biochemical substances associated with pain and inflammation (23):

- pH: Acidic levels in muscles are associated with pain and reduced sensitivity of nociceptors. Acidosis activates acid-sensitive ion channels (ASICs) and vanilloid nociceptors, contributing to hyperalgia.
- Neuropeptides: SP sensitizes nociceptors and elicits inflammatory responses. Calcitonin gene-related peptide (CGRP) modulates nociceptor terminals and may intensify the response to excess ACh.
- Catecholamines: Elevated levels of norepinephrine (NE) and serotonin (5-HT) are found in active MTrPs. 5-HT has pro-nociceptive effects and NE could be related to increased sympathetic activity in MTrPs.
- Cytokines: Elevations of TNF-α, IL-1β, IL-6 and IL-8 are associated with inflammation and pain. These cytokines sensitize nociceptors and have time- and dose-dependent effects. More research is needed to understand the cytokine cascade in muscle pain.

MTrPs are common and complex in non-joint musculoskeletal pain and are often found in asymptomatic individuals. Microanalytical techniques allow direct study of the biochemical environment of MTrPs, revealing elevations of substances related to pain and inflammation. Future research should focus on identifying the mechanisms responsible for MPS in order to develop effective treatments that address these mechanisms and factors perpetuating the syndrome.

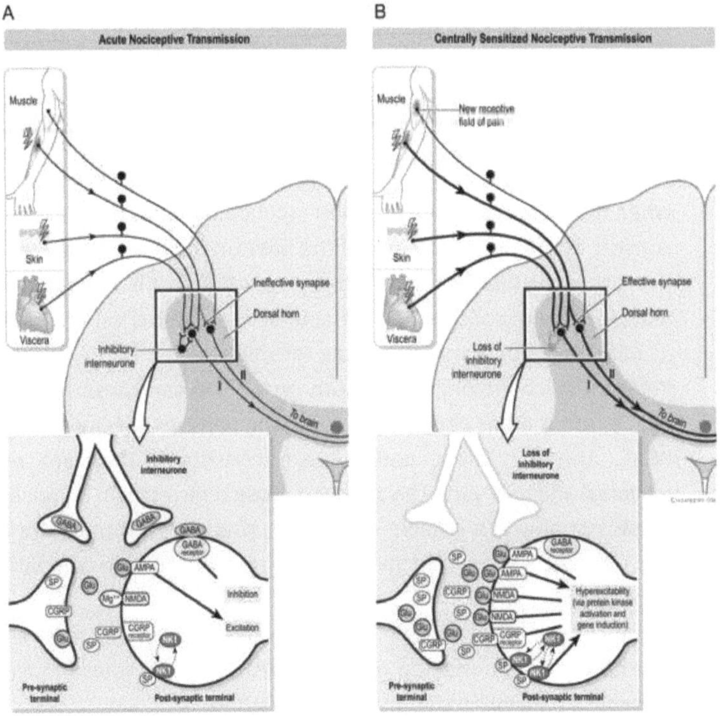

Transition from normal to pathological pain perception via central sensitization in the dorsal horn of the spinal cord. Boxes of central synaptic transmission (A) Acute nociceptive transmission. Nociceptive signals may originate from muscle, skin or visceral afferent neurons. (B) Centrally sensitized nociceptive transmission (23).

2.2. Characteristics of the PGMs.

The following are the key clinical features of myofascial trigger points (MTrPs) that physical therapists should recognize for the diagnosis of myofascial trigger point syndrome (MTS) (24):

- Tension and tight band: Muscles with a PGM feel tight to palpation, especially compared to the healthy opposite side. This tightness is due to the presence of tight bands in the affected muscle. The tight band is a distinctive feature of PGM, although it may be difficult to identify in deep or excess fatty muscles.
- Focality of pain: On palpation of the taut band, a specific point is identified that is noticeably painful, known as the PGM. Moderate

pressure on this point can elicit an intense painful response, known as the jump sign. This sign indicates high sensitivity at the PGM, although its variability and subjectivity make it less reliable in studies, with algometry being a more accurate tool for measuring pain threshold.

- Local twitch response: The local twitch response (REL) is observed when the PGM is pinched or when rapid palpation is performed. It consists of a rapid contraction of the fibers in the tense band, while the rest of the muscle remains relaxed. Although it is an important feature, it is not considered an essential diagnostic criterion due to its difficulty to obtain and variable reliability.
- Referred pain: Prolonged pressure on a PGM can cause referred pain to other areas of the body, following patterns specific to each PGM. Although these patterns are consistent, they are not universal and may vary. The ability to cause referred pain is variable and is not always a reliable diagnostic criterion, with puncture of the TMP being more effective in inducing referred pain compared to palpation.
- Stiffness and shortening: PGMs cause stiffness at rest and shortening of the affected muscle, which can limit joint mobility and cause pain when the muscle is stretched.
- Weakness and pain on contraction: Muscles with PGMs may experience weakness without atrophy, probably due to central inhibition. Electromyography shows that these muscles fatigue more easily and have a slower recovery after exercise. Muscle contraction tends to be more painful when the muscle is shortened.
- Activating mechanism: PGMs can be activated by direct mechanisms (such as trauma or overload) or indirect mechanisms (such as other PGMs, visceral diseases, or stress). Identifying these mechanisms can help in the diagnosis of MDS.

These clinical features are fundamental to the diagnosis and treatment of myofascial trigger points and may vary in presentation between individuals.

2.3. Types of PGMs

Muscle trigger points are hypersensitive areas within a skeletal muscle that, when pressed, cause local pain and often referred pain in other areas of the body. They are classified in various ways according to their activity, origin and clinical behavior. The main types of muscle trigger points are detailed below (25, 26).

2.3.1. According to its activity.

- Active trigger points: They are the direct cause of pain. They are those that cause spontaneous and constant pain, even without pressure or stimulus. These trigger points are the direct cause of the pain and are usually associated with a decrease in the functionality of the affected muscle. When pressed, they reproduce the referred pain and can trigger a muscle spasm response. Active trigger points are responsible for myofascial pain syndrome and can cause significant muscle dysfunction (25, 26).

- Latent trigger points: These do not cause pain unless stimulated by pressure or specific muscle activity. Although they are not painful to the touch in a normal state, they can limit mobility and generate muscle weakness. Latent trigger points can be activated in situations of stress, muscle overuse, injury or fatigue, becoming active trigger points. They are the most common and can remain latent for long periods of time (25, 26).

2.3.2. According to their origin:

- Primary trigger points: They develop independently and have no clear underlying cause. They are directly related to muscle overexertion, overuse, improper posture or trauma. These points are what initially trigger muscle pain and, if left untreated, can contribute to the development of other trigger points in neighboring muscles (25, 26).

- Secondary trigger points: They originate as a result of another condition or dysfunction, such as nerve entrapment, radiculopathy (nerve root irritation) or joint dysfunction. These points usually develop in response to muscle tension generated by the primary condition, and their treatment must include the underlying cause for complete recovery (25, 26).

2.3.3. According to their relationship with other trigger points.

- Satellite trigger points: These develop in areas near a primary trigger point that has been active for a long time without adequate treatment. As the primary trigger point remains active, it can generate excessive tension in nearby muscles, leading to the appearance of these satellite trigger points. It is important to treat both primary and satellite trigger points to achieve complete pain relief (25, 26).

- Associated trigger points: These trigger points are found in muscles that are functionally or biomechanically related to the muscle containing the primary trigger point. Associated trigger points may develop in response to compensatory overload of neighboring muscles in an attempt to relieve pain or dysfunction of the primary affected muscle (25, 26).

   2.3.4. According to the type of pain generated.

- Central PGMs: They are located in the motor plate area of the muscle, where dysfunctional motor plates provoke an energy crisis. This dysfunction generates contraction nodes, which form a nodule within a taut band. These central trigger points are associated with sensitization of local nociceptors in the area, generating pain. It is important to note that these points appear in the region of the muscle where the motor plates, or motor points, are located (25, 26).
- Insertional PGMs: They appear in the areas of muscle insertion, where muscle fibers are anchored to tendons, aponeurosis or bones. The increased tension maintained in these fibers can cause enthesopathy, with inflammation and increased tenderness in the insertion area. This may be more evident in muscles that have sufficient separation between the myotendinous and tenoperiosteal junctions, resulting in the presence of two clearly differentiated insertional PGs (25, 26).

2.4. Mechanism of formation of PGMs.

Myofascial pain can be caused by a variety of factors that may act in isolation or in combination. Understanding these factors is essential to properly address pain and prevent its persistence. The following are the main triggers:

   2.4.1. Triggering factors.

- Acute Trauma: After significant trauma, such as an accident or injury, myofascial pain may occur if pain persists beyond the acute phase of recovery. Under normal circumstances, the pain should subside as the tissue heals. However, when it persists, it is important to consider the possibility of myofascial pain, characterized by trigger points in the affected muscles (27).

- Postural Abnormalities: Postures maintained during daily activities, such as reading, writing or performing work tasks, can induce muscle stress. Poor posture during these activities can cause tension in the muscles and activate trigger points. The accumulation of tension in certain postural positions can lead to the formation of tight bands in the muscles, which in turn can trigger myofascial pain (27).
- Mechanical Factors: Skeletal alterations, such as spinal deviations or joint problems, can cause changes in the muscles that attempt to compensate for these abnormalities. For example, spinal misalignment can result in additional tension in the neck and back muscles, which can activate trigger points and cause pain (27).

- Traffic Accidents: People involved in motor vehicle accidents often suffer from myofascial pain due to the traumatic injuries and strain they experience during impact (28).

2.4.2. Common areas of affectation.

- Head, Neck, Shoulders, Hips and Lumbar Region: These areas are frequently affected by myofascial pain because the muscles in these regions are constantly working against gravity or performing repetitive movements. Muscles that maintain posture or participate in repetitive daily activities are at risk for developing trigger points (28).

2.4.3. Psychological factors.

- Stress and Depression: Prolonged stress and depression can affect muscles by causing prolonged tension. These conditions can trigger trigger points and myofascial pain by altering the way the body handles stress and tension (26).
- Sleep Disturbances: Lack of restful sleep can prevent adequate relaxation of the muscles, causing them to remain in a state of continuous tension. This can lead to the formation of trigger points and myofascial pain, as well as muscle hyperirritability (26).

2.4.4. Nutritional and endocrine factors.

- Nutritional Deficiencies: Deficiencies in essential vitamins, such as B1, B12, C and folic acid, and minerals such as calcium, potassium, iron and magnesium can contribute to the development of trigger points.

Lack of these essential nutrients can affect muscle health and predispose to trigger point formation (26).

- Endocrine Disorders: Problems in thyroid metabolism or other endocrine dysfunctions can affect muscle function and contribute to myofascial pain. Hormonal disturbances may influence the way muscles respond to stress and strain, exacerbating myofascial pain (26).

2.4.5. Degenerative

With age, due to aging muscle tissues may lose elasticity and flexibility, making muscles more prone to develop PGMs. Age-related structural degeneration may also contribute to the formation of these points (28).

2.4.6. Compression of a nerve root.

Compression or irritation of a nerve root can cause sensitization of the corresponding spinal segment and lead to the development of PGMs in the muscles innervated by that nerve root. This may occur due to herniated discs, spinal stenosis or other neurological conditions (28).

2.4.7. Chronic muscular imbalance.

Lack of physical activity can lead to weakening of dynamic muscles, making them more prone to developing PGMs. Inactivity can also contribute to poor posture and muscle imbalances. On the other hand, muscles that are inactive or not used properly can become weak and less efficient, which can lead to compensation by other muscles and the formation of PGMs. Conversely, if the muscles that work to maintain posture become excessively tight and stiff, especially if they are subjected to continuous stress or poor posture, it contributes to the formation of PGMs (28).

Myofascial pain triggers can also become sustained factors if not adequately addressed. Accurate identification and correction of these factors are critical to the effective management of myofascial pain and to prevent recurrence. Addressing not only the current pain, but also the underlying causes, can help eliminate pain and prevent its return.

Maintenance factors

Advanced age
Posture (including at work)
Obesity
Anorexia
Scar tissue (post-surgical)
Sports, leisure, habits
Stress and tension patterns
Metabolic disorders
Disease or disorder
Vitamin deficiencies
Congenital (bone) anomalies
Type of muscle fiber
Direction / orientation of muscle fibers
Muscle shape / morphology (fusiform, etc.)
Psychological factors
Chronicity of trigger points

Table 1. Summary of maintenance factors at PGM points (29).

2.5. Symptoms and physical findings of PGMs.

To understand the origin of myofascial pain, it is essential to know two key concepts, muscle tension and trigger points. Muscle tension arises from the combination of two different factors, viscoelastic tone and contractile activity. Viscoelastic tone can be divided into viscoelastic stiffness and elastic stiffness. Elastic stiffness is related to motion, whereas viscoelastic stiffness is velocity-dependent (25).

Contractile activity is classified into three types: contracture, electrogenic spasm (of pathological origin) and electrogenic rigidity. Contracture does not generate electromyographic activity and originates within the muscle fibers. Electrogenic spasm is a pathological and involuntary muscle contraction initiated in the alpha motor neurons and motor plate. Electrogenic rigidity, on the other hand, refers to muscle tension resulting from contraction in people who are not relaxed (25).

Active PGs cause pain that the patient can identify when pressed, while latent PGs can increase muscle tension and cause shortening without spontaneous pain. Both types of PGs can generate significant motor dysfunction. Active PGs can induce satellite PGs in other muscles, and by treating the key PG, the satellite is often inactivated as well. PGs are commonly activated by muscle overload, whether acute, maintained or repetitive, or by holding the muscle in a shortened position. They can also be activated by nerve compression, disrupting communication between neurons and motor plates (6, 30).

Patients with active PGs often experience diffuse pain in muscles and joints, and the pain may radiate to a distance from the PG. The pain is referred in muscle-specific patterns and sometimes presents as numbness or paresthesia. In addition to pain, PGs can cause alterations in autonomic functions such as excessive sweating and balance problems, as well as muscle weakness and spasm. These dysfunctions can lead to decreased functional capacity and motor coordination (31, 32).

Pain associated with PGs can disrupt sleep, intensifying pain sensitivity the next day. Holding the muscle in a shortened position or under pressure during sleep may increase pain and affect the quality of rest (33).

As for physical findings in a muscle affected by a PG, pain increases with stretching, and a decrease in muscle strength and endurance is also observed. PGs are identified as painful nodules in palpable tight bands within the muscles. The more active the PGs, the more severe the restriction in range of motion and increased muscle tension (6, 30).

On palpation of a superficial muscle, a nodule can be detected in the tense band, extending from the nodule to the muscle insertions. This sign' may reduce or disappear after effective inactivation of the PG. Palpation reveals an extremely tender nodule within the taut band. The pain response may vary with small changes in applied pressure. For recognition, applying pressure to a PG may elicit a referred pain pattern that the patient may recognize as familiar, indicating that the PG is active. This is crucial for diagnosis. In addition to projected pain, PGs can cause hypersensitivity to pressure and dysesthesias (34).

Sudden palpation of a PG often causes a transient spasm in the muscle fibers. This spasm may be similar to that caused by the insertion of a needle. Active PGs reduce the range of passive motion due to pain. This limitation is more pronounced with passive stretching than with active muscle movement. Range of motion usually recovers once the PG is inactivated (35, 36).

When contracting a muscle with an active PG against a fixed resistance, pain intensifies, especially If the muscle is in a shortened position. Muscles with active PGs often show variable weakness between individuals and muscles (35, 36).

Electromyographic (EMG) studies show that these muscles fatigue faster and become exhausted earlier than normal muscles, often due to reflex inhibition triggered by PG (37).

<table><tr><td align="center">**Symptoms of autonomic changes**</td></tr></table>

Hypersalivation: increased saliva.
Epilora: abnormal overflow of tears flowing down the cheeks
Conjunctivitis: eye reddening
Ptosis: eyelid puffiness Blurred vision
Increased nasal secretion.
Goose bumps

Summary of symptoms of autonomic changes (29).

<table><tr><td align="center">**Physical findings**</td></tr></table>

Small nodules about the size of a pinhead.
Pea-sized nodules
Large lumps.
Several large packages side by side.
Soft spots submerged in taut bands of semi-hard muscle that are palpated like a rope.
Rope-like strips arranged side by side like partially cooked spaghetti.
The skin above a trigger point is often slightly warmer than the surrounding skin due to increased metabolic/autonomic activity.

Summary of physical findings (29).

3. EVALUATION AND DIAGNOSIS.

3.1.   Referred pain and tenderness.

Referred pain and hypersensitivity are key to identifying the muscles responsible for myofascial pain syndrome. Patients are often unaware of the trigger point (TP) in the muscle causing the pain, as the pain is often felt in areas away from the TP. Referred pain patterns are predictable and help localize the affected muscle. Myofascial pain is deep and continuous, although it may present as sharp stinging or stabbing. PG-referred pain patterns are usually directed toward the periphery of the body in 85% of cases, while only 10% of the patterns are local. The patterns are useful for localizing the PG, but relying solely on the location of the pain reported by the patient can lead to errors in most cases. For a correct evaluation, the use of trigger point charts is recommended. In addition, when PGs are more active, the pain is more widespread and intense (38).

In pain drawings, solid red areas represent essential areas of pain, while dotted areas show less common areas of pain. A black or white X indicates the frequent location of a PG, although they can be found anywhere in the affected muscle (6, 38).

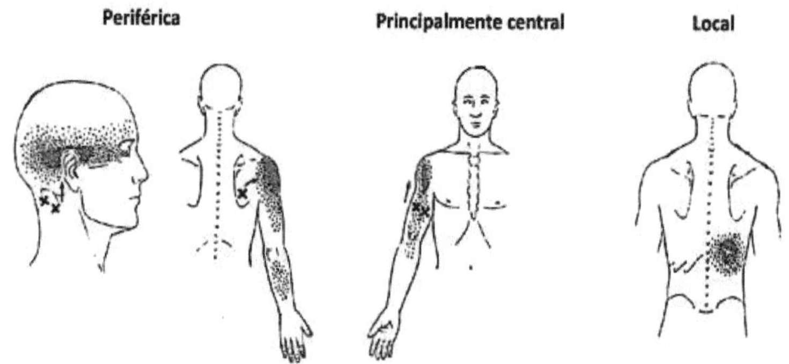

Figure 5. Directions in which PGMs can produce pain (6).

Pain pattern drawing is a useful tool for locating trigger points (TP) responsible for myofascial pain, as patients' verbal descriptions are often inaccurate. Blank body silhouettes are used for the patient or clinician to draw the pain areas, improving communication and diagnostic accuracy.

This graphic recording is essential for comparing the patient's pain patterns with known patterns of individual muscles (6, 38).

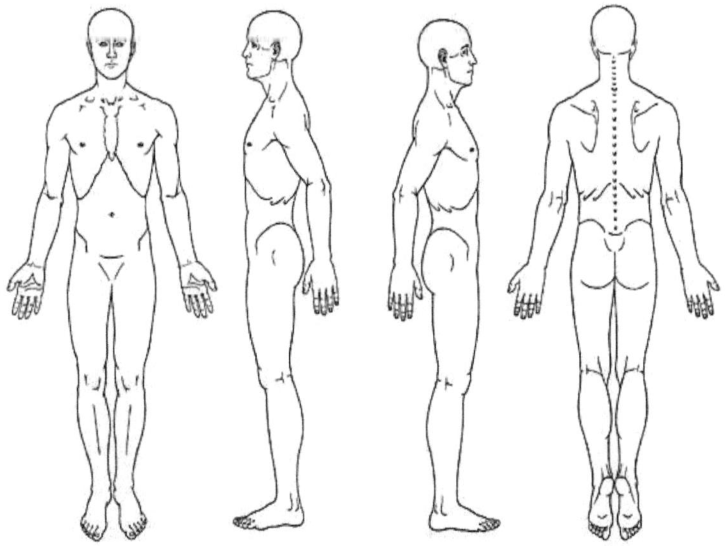

Figure 6. Body silhouette seen in frontal, left and right lateral, as well as posterior for marking the painful area or PGM (6).

The process consists of asking the patient to point to the painful area and having the clinician draw it on the silhouette. The patient then reviews the drawing to make it more accurate. Areas of more intense pain are marked with solid red, while areas of less frequent or less intense pain are dotted. For numbness or tingling, other colors may be used. Trigger points are marked with an X, and after treatment can be marked where it was applied (6, 38).

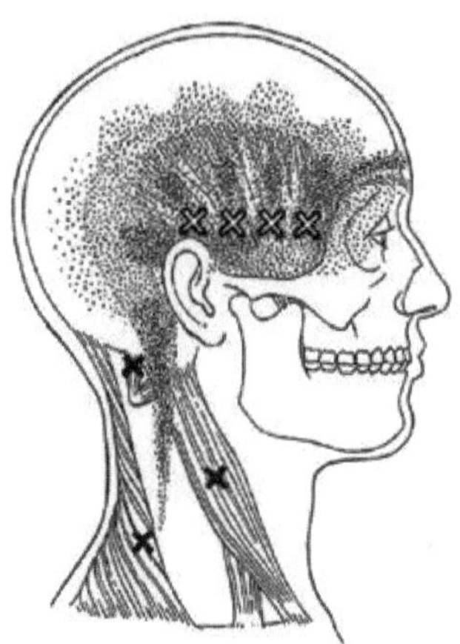

Pain pattern in common tension headache, caused by the superimposition of the referred patterns (dots) of MGP in temporal (white x), suboccipital (superior black x), ECOM (middle black x), and upper trapezius (inferior black x) (6).

Recording these details helps monitor the evolution of the pain and provides a clearer picture of the source of the problem. In addition, comparing the patient's pattern with trigger point charts helps confirm that their pain is real and shared by other patients. This reinforces the patient's confidence and improves the relationship with the clinician. Interpretation of the initial pain patterns is key to determining whether the pain is coming from a myofascial trigger point (TP) from a single muscle or from several overlapping patterns. Myofascial patterns are rarely symmetrical and their extent may increase with PG activity. When several muscles refer pain to the same area, the area may be more painful and hyperaesthetic. For successful treatment, it is important to inactivate all involved PGs (6, 38).

The clinical history should include the evolution of the pain pattern, as a stable pattern suggests a more rapid resolution with appropriate treatment. If the pain has spread to multiple muscles, it is critical to eliminate the perpetuating factors for lasting relief. At follow-up visits, treatment success is measured by comparing previous pain patterns with current pain patterns. If the patient experiences the same pain after treatment, there may be unresolved perpetuating factors. If partial improvement is noted, the pain may have changed location, revealing other active PGs that need to be addressed. Keeping a detailed record of pain patterns is crucial for measuring progress and adjusting treatment (6, 38).

3.2. Medical history.

The initial evaluation of the patient's history and records. Prior to the first consultation, the patient is asked to provide a timeline of important life events. The timeline should include (39, 40, 41, 42).

- The chronology of the patient's life events should include dates and places of residence, studies, marriages, living children (ages and places of residence), sports activities, travel and occupations (type of work, location and employer).
- The chronology of medical history should include illnesses, infections, accidents (fractures, falls, etc.), surgeries, dental procedures, pregnancies and abortions, allergies (testing and desensitization) and vaccinations. It is common for the patient to omit a major accident if there was no fracture, but further questioning may reveal the complete history.
- The patient is usually informed about his or her respiratory allergies, but special attention should be paid to discovering food allergies and symptom-provoking foods. Myofascial trigger points are aggravated by high histamine levels and active allergies. Marking the skin for dermographism is a simple way to identify elevated histamine levels. In the case of respiratory allergies, it is helpful to reduce exposure by electrostatic air purifiers. However, simply owning one may not be enough. One patient reported using it every night, but on digging a little deeper, she revealed that she also kept her windows open throughout the night, which allowed pollen to enter, neutralizing the effectiveness of the purifier.
- The medication list should include all current drugs, including vitamin and mineral supplements. The patient should be asked to bring a bottle of each medication to confirm the exact dosage of prescription medications, over-the-counter medications, and nutritional supplements. It is also essential to make a list of medications taken in the past that have caused side effects or have not been effective in relieving pain.

The patient should be asked to send a copy of all available medical records prior to the consultation and request all outstanding reports from previous physicians, especially orthopedic or neurological consultation reports. These documents should be carefully reviewed prior to the first visit.

3.3.   Patient interview

During history taking, the patient's comfort should be ensured by teaching him/her the principles of good body posture. If necessary, a footrest can be provided for patients whose legs do not reach the floor well, if the elbows do not reach the armrests of the chair, these should be raised, a cushion can also be used to correct the inclination of the body caused by pelvic asymmetry. Placing a small pillow in the lumbar hollow helps to maintain correct posture without effort, making it easier for the patient to sit upright instead of slouching forward (39, 40, 41, 42).

Patients are often surprised to discover the immediate relief they can feel by reducing the muscle tension caused by these mechanical factors. This relief helps them understand the significant impact these factors have on their pain. To protect against the cold, a towel or scarf can be provided to cover the patient's shoulders. If their hands or feet are cold, applying dry heat to the abdomen helps to warm the central core of the body and improve blood circulation to the extremities. Often, precise postural and environmental corrections allow the patient to tolerate a prolonged 30- to 45-minute consultation without additional discomfort (39, 40, 41, 42).

It is essential to establish empathy with the patient in order to properly understand his or her medical history. Empathy involves putting oneself in the patient's shoes and objectively understanding the patient's life problems, including work, personal relationships, and emotional stresses. However, it is important not to identify emotionally with the patient, as this can negatively affect the patient-physician relationship and damage the physician's mental health (39, 40, 41, 42).

If the pain is constant and affects multiple areas, the patient may say "it hurts all over", or concentrate on the area of greatest pain, omitting to mention other areas until the main pain has been relieved. It is essential to learn to discriminate the areas of actual pain. For example, one patient described pain in her "TMJ," but when pointing to the location, she placed her finger on the mastoid process behind the ear, and she had never had pain in the temporomandibular joint. A brief review of the major body systems ensures that no significant problems have been overlooked. When checking the gastrointestinal system, ask about a history of diarrhea, constipation, nausea, heartburn, abdominal pain, hemorrhoids, and blood in the stool, among others. Patients with low folate levels often experience intermittent diarrhea with explosive bowel movements. Constipation is often related to hypothyroidism or vitamin B1 deficiency. If patients report poor sleep, it is important to inquire if they have difficulty falling asleep, if they wake up frequently during the night, or if they wake up too early and cannot get back to sleep. The cause of the sleep disruption, such as a chronic urinary tract infection or prostate problem, should also be investigated (39, 40, 41, 42).

3.4. Examination of the patient.

The dysfunctions and phenomena associated with trigger points are discussed. It is assumed that the clinician has reviewed the patient's complete medical history and performed a detailed neurological examination to distinguish between neurological and myofascial symptoms. Here we differentiate between primary effects, derived from the physiology of the PGM, and secondary effects, induced by its activity. It is crucial to understand that each patient is unique and there is no universal solution for musculoskeletal pain (43, 44).

It is essential to observe the patient's posture and movements while walking, sitting or performing daily tasks. Patients with active PGMs tend to move slowly, avoiding movements that may cause muscle pain. Key observations include, symmetrical use of arms and hands, body rotations and spontaneous stretching movements. These signs can indicate which muscles are affected. Limitation of mobility is a direct effect of increased muscle tension caused by PGMs, and is augmented by pain from sensitized nociceptors. Reflex weakness may arise from PGM-induced inhibition, affecting both the affected muscle and related muscles. Some patients have poor muscle coordination, complicating treatment, while athletes can regain function quickly with appropriate treatment. A muscle with active PGs is functionally shortened and weakened. Attempting to stretch it causes pain before reaching normal range. This painful restriction can be identified with global mobility testing. In addition, latent PGMs, common in the elderly, limit movement without obvious pain, but can be effectively treated with myofascial therapy and stretching (43, 44).

It is important not to assume that muscle weakness only requires strengthening exercises. PGM-induced weakness can be detected by static and dynamic strength testing. Static tests rely on cortical control, while dynamic tests monitor functional tasks requiring coordination, controlled by the cerebellum. In cases of weakness, treatment involves inactivation of the responsible PGs and motor re-education of the patient. Referred pain sensitivity is closely related to referred pain from a neurophysiological perspective. Research suggests that by stimulating the PGM, pain can be elicited both at the site of the PGM and in areas away from the PGM, called referral zones. One key study observed that, when pressure was applied to active MMPs, not only did local and referred pain occur, but pain thresholds in the cutaneous, subcutaneous and intramuscular areas decreased significantly in both the MMP area and the pain reference zone. This suggests that PGMs, active or latent, may reduce pain thresholds, being more marked in active PGs (43, 44).

Tenderness in the referral areas appears to correlate with irritability of PGs, implying an interaction between these points and surrounding areas. Furthermore, other studies have corroborated these findings, highlighting that referred pain and hypersensitivity to stimulation are common in multiple tissue layers, contributing to the complexity of pain associated with PGs. It is crucial to differentiate this phenomenon from other types of hypersensitivity such as enthesopathy, which is limited to areas of muscle insertion, whereas trigger point pain is more diffusely distributed (43, 44).

3.5. Diagnose a PGM.

Criteria for diagnosing myofascial pain syndrome vary among investigations, but the most common are (39, 45):

- The presence of a painful nodule in a tense and palpable muscle band.
- Reproduction of pain when pressing the myofascial trigger point. Myofascial pain syndrome is often confused with fibromyalgia.

According to the 1990 American College of Rheumatology (ACR) criteria, fibromyalgia is diagnosed based on (25 46, 47):

- Chronic generalized pain above and below the waist, lasting more than three months.
- The presence of 11 of 18 established pain points. Recently, the 2010 criteria of the same institution have been published. Frequently, patients with fibromyalgia present with secondary myofascial trigger points. However, there is a clear clinical distinction between the two conditions, which is crucial, as the treatments are different.

3.5.1. Exploration of the PGMs.

Accurate identification of MMPs is key to diagnosing and treating myofascial pain. The following is a description of how to perform the exploration of MMPs and the associated diagnostic criteria (6, 44, 48).

The first step is to identify which muscles to explore based on the patient's range of motion limitations and referred pain patterns. The examiner can resist a movement to contract the suspected muscle and palpate it to confirm its location. It is essential that the patient be in a comfortable, relaxed position in a comfortable temperature environment. The muscle must be completely relaxed, since, if it is tense, it will be difficult to distinguish the tense bands associated with PGs from normal muscle fibers (6, 48).

Careful palpation is key to locating tight bands and nodules associated with PGs. There are three main palpation techniques (6, 44, 48):

- Flat palpation: It is used for superficial muscles, where it is palpated perpendicularly to the muscle fibers. It is a technique used to explore muscles that are only accessible from one side, such as the infraspinatus. This method makes it possible to detect tight bands within the muscle through the movement of the skin and the perception of changes in the muscle fibers. The procedure used is described in the figure below:

Initiating palpation (Figure A), the examiner pushes the skin to one side so that it is mobilized over the muscle to be examined. This initial mobilization of the skin facilitates access to the underlying muscle fibers. Sliding the fingertip (Figure B), with the skin displaced, the fingertip slides transversely to the muscle fibers, allowing detection of the taut bands. These bands are felt as chordal structures rolling under the finger. The texture of these taut bands is firmer than that of normal muscle fibers. Finishing the movement (Figure C), at the end of the sliding across the muscle fibers, the skin is pushed to the other side, thus completing the palpation path. This maneuver not only makes it possible to identify the tight bands, but also to locate the point where the greatest pain is concentrated on pressure, corresponding to the trigger point. When this technique is performed more vigorously and quickly, it is known as sudden palpation, which can intensify the perception of tight bands and their diagnosis.

- Pincer palpation: Used when the muscle can be grasped between the fingers, such as the sternocleidomastoid. The following is a description of the procedure used in the figure below: Pincer palpation (Figure A), the muscle fibers of the muscle in question are grasped between the thumb and triphalangeal fingers, forming a pincer that allows the tension within the muscle to be captured. The tight band and trigger point are in this area. Perception of the taut band (Figure B), by pressing and letting the muscle fibers roll between the fingers, the hardness of the taut band is felt. The change in angle of the distal phalanges creates a rocking motion that enhances sensitivity and discrimination, helping to detect the stiff texture of the taut band and any fine details. Escaping from the fingers (Figure C), the palpable edge of the taut band is defined when it escapes from between the fingertips, which can often elicit a local twitch response. This phenomenon is characteristic of active trigger points.
- Deep palpation: For deep muscles where the previous techniques are not feasible.

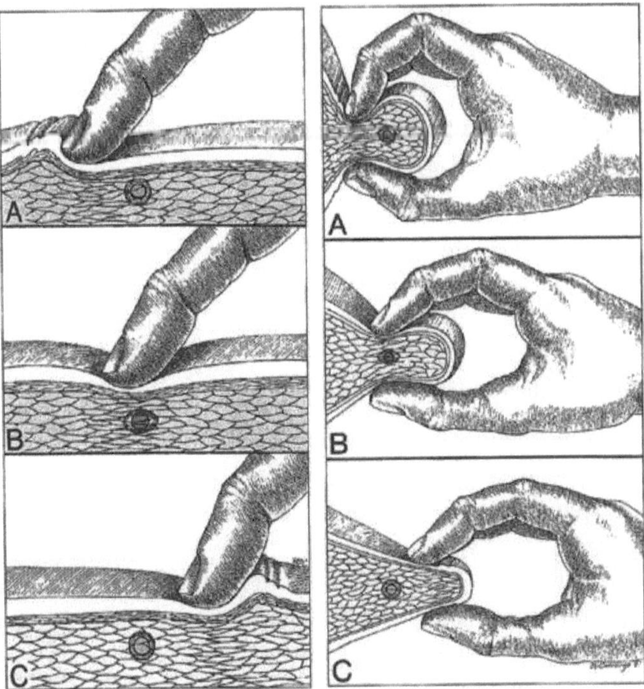

Figure 8. The image on the left shows the flat palpation of a tense band and its PGM. In the image on the right we find a pincer palpation of a tense band at the level of a PGM (6).

The examiner's fingernails should be short to avoid causing unnecessary pain to the patient, which could interfere with the correct identification of PGMs. Long nails may cause cutaneous pain to be mistaken for actual PG pain (6, 44, 48).

Although the use of dermometers (to measure skin conductance) has been suggested as a tool to detect PGMs, these devices are not sufficiently reliable. Further studies would be needed to evaluate their efficacy and reliability. The most reliable feature for diagnosing a PGM is the presence of exquisite pain on palpation of a nodule in a palpable tense band of muscle. If pressure on this nodule reproduces the patient's characteristic pain, the PGM is considered active. Other indicators, such as limitation in range of motion and local spasm response, also support the diagnosis (6, 44, 48).

PGMs can be difficult to detect, especially in deep muscles, and excessive pressure can trigger an exaggerated response in the patient, known as the "jump sign". To obtain a quantitative assessment of pain on pressure, an algometer can be used (6, 44, 48).

3.5.2. Complementary explorations: imaging techniques.

Currently, there are no widely accepted laboratory tests or imaging techniques to diagnose trigger points (TP). Diagnosis of myofascial pain syndrome remains predominantly clinical, although tools have recently been developed to help confirm the presence of PGs, with needle electromyography and ultrasonography being particularly promising for clinical use.

- Needle electromyography: This was initially explored in 1957 and was later found to detect electromyographic activity specific to myofascial PGs. Animal and human studies have confirmed the presence of characteristic activity, such as motor plate "noise" and high-voltage spikes, which are indicative of, but not exclusive to, PGs. Surface electromyography shows how PGs affect normal muscle function, increasing reactivity, delaying relaxation and causing increased fatigue. Recent research has used computer analysis to study how PGs influence muscle activity, revealing that they can affect motor function locally and in related muscles via the central nervous system. It has been observed that PGs can cause spasm in referred muscles and that some muscles tend to develop PGs in response to spasm in other muscles. This suggests a complex interaction between PG-affected muscles and their influence on the activity of other muscles. In addition, the presence of PGs may induce an abnormal motor reaction in nearby muscles. Finally, the ability of PGs to cause inhibition in muscle function can significantly alter normal muscle performance, and restoration of normal patterns may require re-education of the affected muscle. These phenomena suggest that motor dysfunction caused by PGs is as complex as sensory dysfunction and deserves further investigation (23, 36, 49).
- Ultrasonography: It was first used by Michael Margolis to visualize the PG response. This technique can complement electromyographic recordings and has potential to be an effective diagnostic tool for PGs, although its application requires skill in palpation or insertion of a needle into the PG to elicit the expected response. The use of a 12.5

MHz transducer over a muscle band has shown a focused hypoechoic zone of 0.16 ± 0.11 cm², which has previously been identified as a myofascial trigger point. This zone does not appear in healthy muscle tissue or around other trigger points. Another study performed with a 7-12 MHz transducer on the anterior rectus also revealed changes in echogenicity in areas previously associated with myofascial trigger points. When using an ultrasound with a 5-12 MHz transducer, a higher frequency of local contractile response was observed when stimulating a trigger point, compared to clinical observation. This contraction was associated with a better response to treatment. However, in this study, no imaging abnormalities were found to correspond to myofascial trigger points, something that also occurred in another study with few patients. The cost of ultrasonography equipment has decreased considerably, while the quality of the images has improved. In our center, we have found hypoechoic areas with similar characteristics to those described by other authors that correlate clinically with myofascial trigger points. However, when interpreting these studies it is important to consider variables such as the characteristics of the equipment, the transducer, the operator's training, the patient's evolution time and the previous use of infiltrations (50, 51, 52, 53).

- Elastography, ultrasound and MRI: The use of imaging techniques such as elastography, ultrasound and MRI has allowed a more accurate assessment of myofascial trigger points (MTrPs). These tools help identify structural and functional changes in muscle tissue that are not always evident by traditional physical examination.

- Elastography has been shown to be effective in detecting increased muscle stiffness in areas affected by MMPs. Both ultrasound elastography and magnetic resonance elastography can identify and quantify the characteristic tight bands of PGMs, differentiating them from healthy tissue. These techniques allow a noninvasive and detailed assessment of changes in muscle elasticity, which facilitates the diagnosis and follow-up of patients (54, 55, 56).

- Ultrasound is another key tool in the evaluation of MMPs, especially to detect alterations in the structure and echogenicity of muscle tissue. Ultrasound imaging makes it possible to observe differences in muscle texture, such as hyperechogenic areas, which correspond to the areas where PGMs are located. In addition, its ability to visualize the tissue in real time makes it useful for guiding therapeutic interventions (57, 58, 59).

- On the other hand, magnetic resonance imaging (MRI) offers a deeper and more detailed view of the muscles affected by MMPs. It makes it possible to identify not only structural changes in the muscle, but also to evaluate the surrounding tissue, which is particularly useful in deeper or complex muscle areas. MRI complements ultrasound by providing higher resolution images for accurate diagnosis of PGMs (60, 61, 62).

Overall, these imaging technologies have proven to be valuable tools for improving the diagnosis and treatment of myofascial trigger points, providing objective information about alterations in muscle tissue structure and function. This facilitates a more accurate approach to treatment planning in patients with myofascial pain.

- Algometry: Measures pain sensitivity using pressure or electrical stimulation. Three types of information it provides have been identified (34, 63, 64).
  - Local pain threshold: The pressure required for pain to be initiated at a specific point.
  - Referred pain threshold: The pressure that causes pain in areas distant from the point of application.
  - Pain tolerance: The maximum pressure the patient can withstand before the pain becomes intolerable.

The spring algometer, designed in 1986 and widely used since then, measures these thresholds by applying pressure to the skin using a calibrated circular tip. The measurement is made in Kg or Newtons, and the accuracy depends on the diameter of the algometer tip. This instrument is useful for comparing pain sensitivity before and after treatments. However, it has limitations such as, it does not determine the cause of the pain, which can be myofascial, fibromyalgia, bursitis, etc. The measurement can be affected by tissue thickness and muscle sensitivity. The technique requires dexterity and correct localization of the point of maximum sensitivity. Recent research has shown that algometry may not clearly distinguish between active and latent trigger points, and that results may vary depending on the pressure applied. Although useful for research and clinical purposes, it should be interpreted with caution (34, 63, 64).

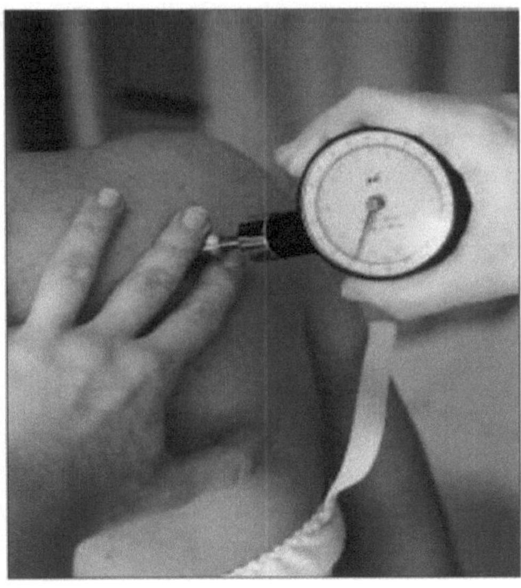

Pressure measurement using the algometer on a PGM in the infraspinatus muscle (34).

- Thermography: Using infrared radiometry or liquid crystal films, it measures changes in skin temperature. Electronic thermography is more accurate and convenient, showing thermal variations that can indicate problems such as myofascial trigger points. However, a thermal change does not always indicate a trigger point, as it may be caused by other conditions such as radiculopathy or local inflammation. Studies have found that the skin temperature over a trigger point may be higher, but this does not always translate into accurate trigger point detection. Studies also show that active trigger points can cause hyperthermia in the skin, while mechanical stimulation can cause "reflex" hypothermia. Thermography can identify hot areas, but it can also have false positives and negatives. Combining thermography with other methods, such as palpation and algometric measurement, improves the accuracy of trigger point identification. However, interpretation of the results should be done with caution and complemented with other diagnostic evaluations (65, 66, 67, 68).

So far, the literature has not addressed some key questions about the thermal changes associated with trigger points (TP). Since many acupuncturists employ devices to measure skin resistance to identify the optimal place to insert the needle and treat a PG or sore spot, it would be of great interest to conduct a blinded study to investigate the region of a hot spot and look for points of low resistance. It would be useful to determine how often these low resistance points coincide with hot spots and whether these points have a PG (active or latent) nearby. PG identification should be based on accurate diagnostic criteria applied by evaluators with high interexaminer reliability. Furthermore, since several studies have shown that PG dysfunction is influenced by sympathetic nervous system activity, investigating how PGs affect sympathetic control of cutaneous perfusion could enrich our understanding of the relationship between myofascial PGs and the autonomic nervous system.

4. LOCALIZATION AND REFERRED PAIN OF TRIGGER POINTS IN UPPER LIMBS.

It is essential to understand the function and characteristics of each muscle, as well as its relationship to pain and myofascial trigger points (MTrPs). Next, the musculature of the head, face, neck, trunk, shoulder, arm, forearm and hand will be explored in detail. Addressing their origin, insertion and action, which we will use the different treatises of anatomy atlases (69, 70, 71, 72, 73), as well as the symptoms associated with referred pain and the presence of MMPs (29, 74). We will also discuss possible causes of muscle dysfunctions, differential diagnosis that allows identification of related problems, and offer recommendations and effective techniques for treatment (75, 76, 77, 78, 79, 80). This comprehensive approach will provide a clear and practical understanding that will be of great use to both students and professionals in the health care field.

4.1. Musculature of the head and face.

4.1.1. Epicranium (occipitofrontal).

- Occipital:
  - Origin: Lateral part of the two thirds of the superior nuchal line and the mastoid process of the temporal bone.
  - Insertion: Epicranial aponeurosis.
- Front:
  - Origin: Superficial layer of the scalp fascia.
  - Insertion: Epicranial aponeurosis, skin of the eyebrows and base of the nose.
- Actions: When both muscles act in concert, they stretch the scalp backward and upward, raise the eyebrows and generate forehead creases. If only the frontalis muscle is contracted, it raises the eyebrow on the same side.
- Referred pain and PGM:

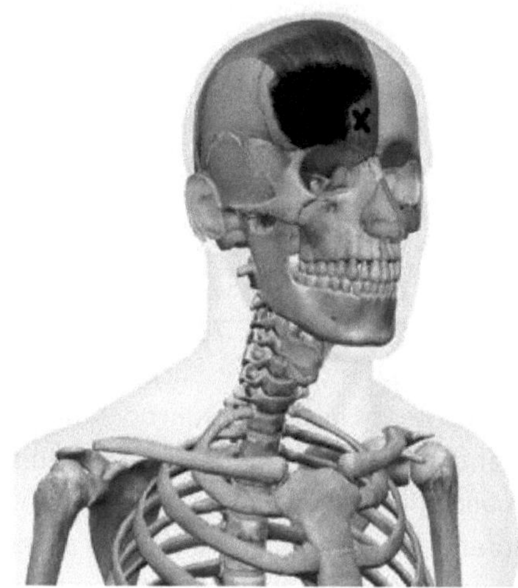

Frontal referred pain areas, marked with black area and PGM marked with black cross.

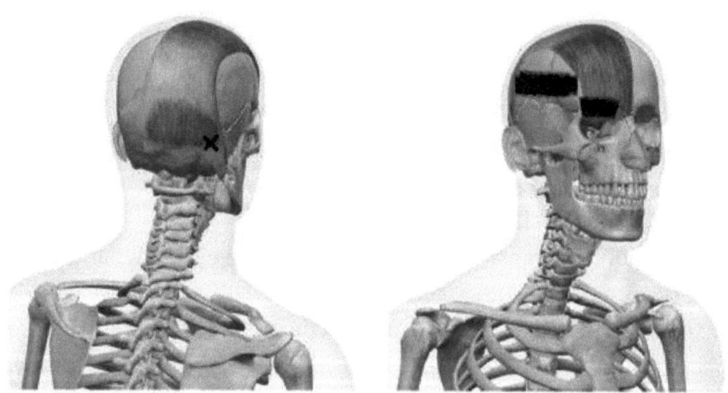

Occipital referred pain areas, marked with black area and PGM marked with black cross.

- Symptoms: Trigger points in the frontalis muscle cause pain in the forehead, over the eyebrow on the same affected side. Trigger points in the occipital muscle cause deep pain in the eye and side of the head, as well as discomfort when resting the head on a pillow.
- Possible causes:
  - Stress or anxiety.

- Ocular problems.
- Differential diagnosis:
  - Compression of the occipital nerve (more superficial).
  - Conditions in other muscles that produce similar pain: temporalis, sternocleidomastoid, splenius, longissimus longissimus of the head, semispinatus, suboccipitalis, trapezius, orbicularis oculi, masseter.
- Recommendations: Avoid furrowing the brow.
- Recommended techniques: Injections, dry needling and PGM release.

4.1.2. Orbicularis oculi.

- Orbital part:
  - Origin: Nasal portion of the frontal bone, frontal process of the maxilla, and internal palpebral ligament.
  - Insertion: Skin of the eyebrow, fusing with neighboring muscles.
- Palpebral part:
  - Origin: Internal palpebral ligament and frontal bone.
  - Insertion: External palpebral raphe.
- Tear part:
  - Origin: Lacrimal fascia and lacrimal bone.
  - Insertion: Tarsus of the eyelids, forming the external palpebral raphe.
- Shares:
  - The orbital part is in charge of closing the eye intensely.
  - The palpebral part gently closes the eye, intervening in blinking and protective closure.
  - The lacrimal part dilates the tear ducts to accumulate tears and compresses the lacrimal sac during blinking.
- Referred pain and PGM:

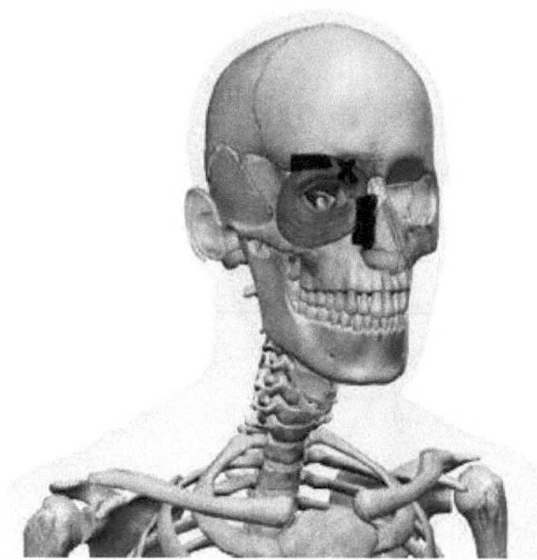

Figure 12. Referred pain represented with black color and trigger point represented with black cross of the orbicularis oculi muscle of the right eye.

- Symptoms: The referred pain is localized in the eyebrow and the side of the nose on the same affected side, extending in some cases to the upper lip and cheek near the nose. Patients may also experience difficulty reading, reporting that letters "jump" or "dance".
- Possible causes:
  - Eye problems such as astigmatism (from squinting).
  - Photophobia.
  - Differential Diagnosis
  - Palpebral ptosis.
  - Migraine.
  - Ocular problems.
  - Affection in other muscles that generate similar pain: occipitofrontal, sternocleidomastoid, zygomatic.
- Recommendations: Check eyesight regularly. Increase the period of rest or sleep. Interrupt fixed gaze such as driving, looking at computer screens, cell phones, etc.
- Recommended techniques: Injections, dry needling and PGM release.

4.1.3. Masseter.

- Origin: Zygomatic arch and maxillary process of the zygomatic bone, in addition to the zygomatic process of the upper jaw.
- Insertion: Branch of the mandible and mandibular angle.
- Actions: Elevates the mandible, facilitating chewing, and moves it forward (protrusion). However, the deeper fibers of the muscle retract the mandible.
- Symptoms: The referred pain appears in the area of the temporomandibular joint, eyebrow, malar bone, mandibular ramus and teeth. It can also cause deep pain in the ear. These trigger points cause joint dysfunction and tooth sensitivity to hot or cold stimuli. In addition, the patient may experience tinnitus.
- Referred pain and PGM:
    - Superficial masseter (Fig. A, B, C)
    - Deep masseter (Fig. D)

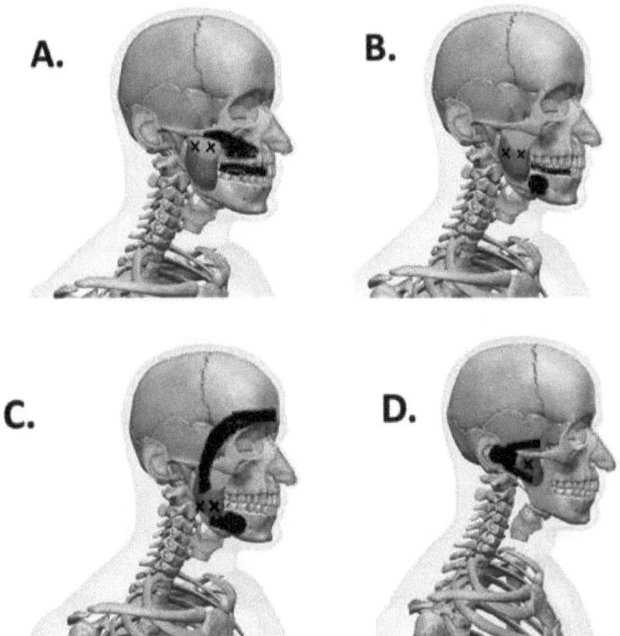

Figure 13. Referred pain represented by black color and PGM of the superficial and deep masseter, represented by black cross.

- Possible causes:
  - Keeping the mouth open for long periods of time (e.g., at the dentist).
  - Surgeries.
  - Overuse of the temporomandibular joint (chewing gum, ice).
  - Bruxism.
  - Stress and anxiety.
- Differential diagnosis
  - Temporomandibular joint dysfunction.
  - Sinusitis.
  - Tinnitus of neurological origin.
  - Dental problems.
  - Arthritis.
- Affection in other muscles with similar referred pain: buccinator, occipitofrontal, temporal, platysma, sternocleidomastoid, head longissimus, semispinal, suboccipital, pterygoid.
- Recommendations: Do not grind the teeth (occlusal splints). Head-neck-tongue posture. No chewing, biting gum, ice cream or nails.
- Recommended techniques: Spraying and stretching, injections, dry needling and PGM release.

4.1.4. Temporary.

- Origin: Fossa of the temporal bone and deep part of the temporal fascia.
- Insertion: Coronoid process and anterior border of the mandibular ramus.
- Shares:
  - Raise the jaw to close the mouth (biting action).
  - The posterior fibers retract the mandible.
- Symptoms: Anterior trigger points generate referred pain in the forehead, just above the eyebrow and in the temple, as well as affecting the upper incisors and canines on the same side. Patients may also feel pain behind the eye. Posterior trigger points cause pain above the ear, in the temporomandibular joint and in the upper molars on the same side. The pain is accompanied by hypersensitivity to touch and dental hypersensitivity.

- Referred pain and PGM:

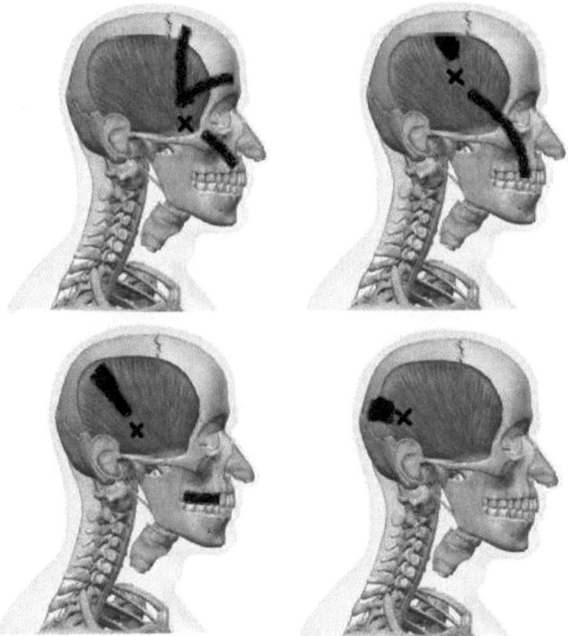

Figure 14. Referred pain represented by black color and myofascial trigger points of the temporalis represented by black cross.

- Possible causes:
    - Temporomandibular joint dysfunctions.
    - Direct trauma.
    - Bruxism.
    - Prolonged immobilization of the jaw (as in dental procedures).
    - Infections or inflammations.
    - Stress and/or anxiety.
    - Differential Diagnosis
    - Dental problems.
    - Migraine.
    - Temporal tendinopathy.
- Affections in other muscles with similar referred pain: platysma, sternocleidomastoid, splenius, longissimo of the head, semispinous,

suboccipital, trapezius, occipitofrontal, buccinator, masseter, pterygoid.
- Recommendations: Chewing gum or hard substances. Tongue position, Air conditioning in car or work. Correct head posture, forward posture. Stretching.
- Recommended techniques: Spraying and stretching, injections, dry needling and PGM release.

4.1.5. Lateral pterygoid

- Origin:
  - Superior fascicle: greater wing of the sphenoid, on its infratemporal aspect.
  - Inferior fascicle: lateral pterygoid plate of the sphenoid.
- Insertion: Inserts into the pterygoid fossa, the neck of the mandible, and the capsule and disc of the temporomandibular joint.
- Functions: During mouth opening, this muscle pulls the mandibular condyle forward, along with the articular disc. In conjunction with the medial pterygoid, it deflects the mandible to the opposite side.
- Referred pain and PGM:

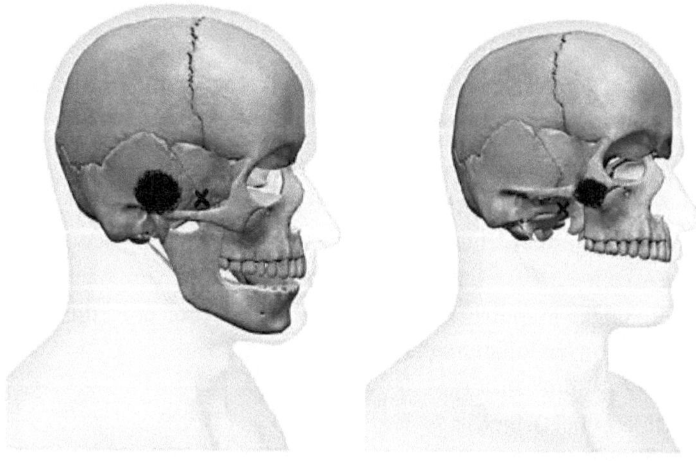

Figure 15. Referred pain represented by black color and PGM of the lateral pterygoid represented by black cross.

- Symptoms: Referred pain in the area of the temporomandibular joint and zygomatic arch. Difficulty and discomfort when chewing and opening the mouth. In some cases, tinnitus (ringing in the ears) may occur.

- Possible causes
  - Keeping the mouth open for prolonged periods of time (e.g. at the dentist).
  - Surgeries.
  - Excessive use of the temporomandibular joint (such as chewing gum or ice).
  - Bruxism (teeth grinding).
  - Stress and anxiety.
- Differential diagnosis
  - Temporomandibular joint dysfunction.
  - Trigeminal neuralgia.
  - Conditions in other muscles with similar referred pain: medial pterygoid, masseter, buccinator, temporalis, platysma.
- Recommendations: Chew on both sides of the mouth. Avoid chewing gum or nail biting. Dental protector, posture of holding the phone between shoulder and neck.
- Recommended techniques: Spraying and stretching, injections and PGM release.

4.1.6. Medial pterygoid.

- Origin: Sphenoid bone, palatine bone and tuberosity of the maxilla.
- Insertion: Branch of the mandible and mandibular foramen.
- Functions: This muscle elevates the mandible for mastication and also participates in mandibular protrusion. Together with the lateral pterygoid, it deflects the mandible to the opposite side.
- Referred pain and PGM:

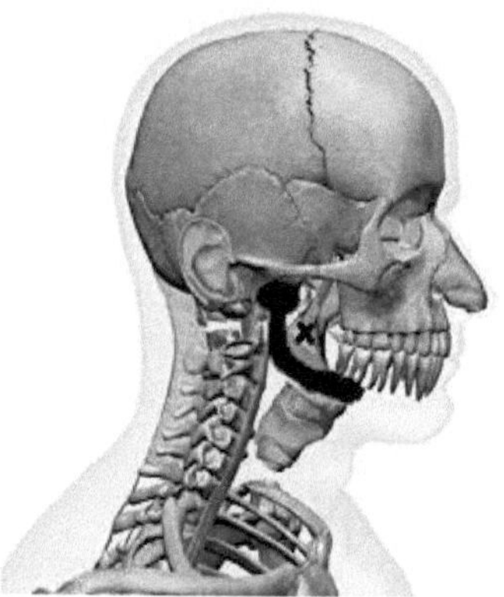

Figure 16. Referred pain represented by black color and PGM of the medial pterygoid represented by black cross.

- Symptoms: Referred pain in the temporomandibular joint area, which may radiate to the clavicle and throat. Pain and difficulty in opening the mouth is experienced.
- Possible causes:
  - Keeping the mouth open for a prolonged period of time (e.g. at the dentist).
  - Surgeries.
  - Excessive use of the temporomandibular joint (such as chewing gum or ice).
  - Bruxism.
  - Stress and anxiety.
  - Arthritis.
- Differential diagnosis:
  - Temporomandibular joint dysfunction.
  - Throat pathologies.
  - Conditions in other muscles with similar referred pain: masseter, temporalis, platysma, lateral pterygoid.
- Recommendations: Head posture. Chewing on both sides of the mouth. Dental protector (soft). Avoid chewing gum or nail biting.
- Recommended techniques: Spraying and stretching, injections and PGM release.

4.1.7. Digastric.

- Anterior portion:
  - Origin: Diastric fossa of the mandible.
  - Insertion: Hyoid bone.
- Posterior portion:
  - Origin: Temporal bone.
  - Insertion: Hyoid bone.
  - Both portions are connected through an intermediate tendon, which attaches to the hyoid bone.
- Functions: This muscle intervenes in the elevation of the hyoid during swallowing, as well as in the depression and retrusion of the mandible.
- Referred pain and PGM:

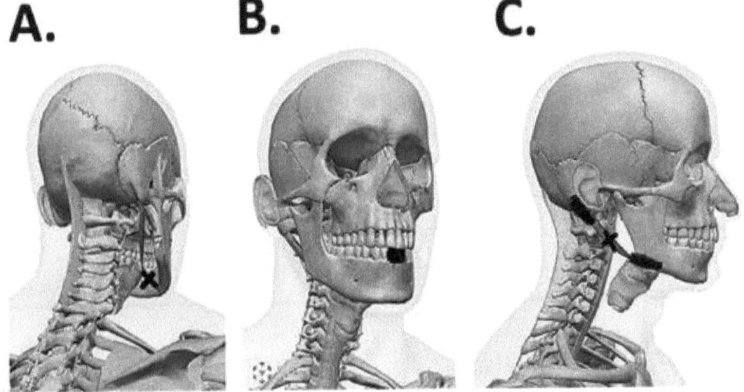

Figure 17. Referred pain represented by black color and PGM of the anterior (represented in figure A and B) and posterior (figure C) portion of the digastric muscle represented by black cross.

- Symptoms:
  - The anterior portion produces pain referred to the four lower incisors, the tongue and, occasionally, the chin.
  - The posterior portion causes pain in the lateral area of the throat, below the pinna, and even in the scalp. Sometimes the patient only experiences difficulty in swallowing, as if there is a lump in the throat, without obvious pain.

- Possible causes:
  - Bruxism.
  - Altered posture with jaw forward.
  - Dysfunction of synergistic muscles, such as the masseter muscles.
  - Prolonged mouth breathing (from keeping the mouth open for a long time).
- Differential diagnosis:
  - Dental problems.
  - Thyroid pathologies.
  - Alterations in the hyoid bone.
  - Conditions in other muscles with similar referred pain: sternocleidomastoid, semispinous, trapezius, masseter, suboccipital.
- Recommendations: Breathing patterns, bruxism, head postures.
- Recommended techniques: Spraying and stretching, injections, and PGM release.

4.2. Musculature of the neck and trunk.

4.2.1. Anterior, middle and posterior scalenes.

- Anterior scalene:
  - Origin: costo-transverse processes of the C3 to C6 vertebrae.
  - Insertion: First rib.
- Middle scalene:
  - Origin: costo-transverse processes of the C2 to C7 vertebrae.
  - Insertion: First rib, and in some cases, also in the second rib.
- Posterior scalene:
  - Origin: costo-transverse processes of the C4 to C6 vertebrae.
  - Insertion: Second rib, and occasionally in the third rib.
- Functions: Working together, these muscles generate a slight flexion of the cervical spine. Unilaterally, they cause a homolateral tilt. In addition, they contribute to inspiration during respiration if the spine acts as a fixed point. They also act as lateral stabilizers of the middle and lower cervical spine.

- Fascial pain and PGM:

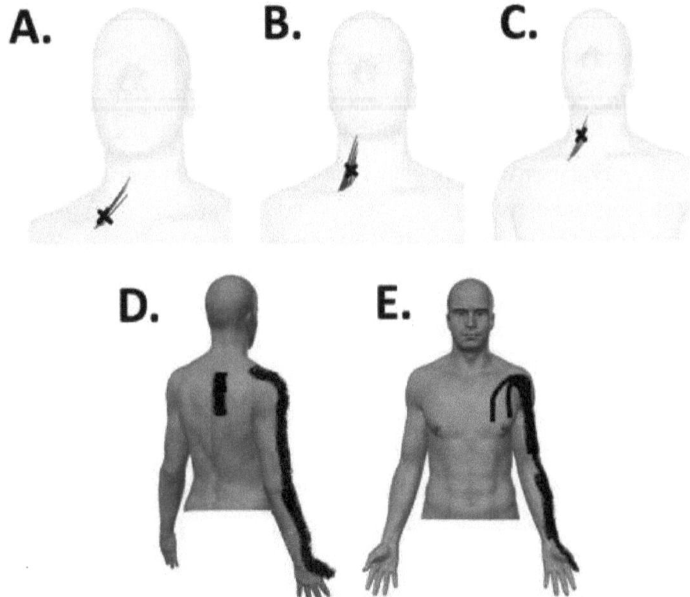

Figure 18. PGM of the anterior (depicted in Figure A), middle (Figure B) and posterior (Figure C) portions of the scalene muscle represented by black cross and referred pain depicted in black color of posterior view (Figure D) and anterior view (Figure E).

- Symptoms: Pain referred to the arm in the lateral part and to the first and second fingers of the hand. There may also be pain in the pectoral region, specifically in the nipple area, and posterior pain in the scapular area. Symptoms include signs of brachial plexus compression.
- Possible causes:
  - Incorrect posture with the head forward.
  - Stress and anxiety (main factors).
  - Respiratory problems such as colds.
  - Differential diagnosis
  - Compression of the brachial plexus.
  - Carpal tunnel syndrome.
  - Cervical disc pathologies.
  - Vascular compression.

- Conditions in other muscles with similar referred pain: subclavian, pectoralis, trapezius, angularis scapulae, supraspinatus, infraspinatus, rhomboid, serratus posterior superior, iliocostalis dorsi, brachioradialis, extensor pollicis, pronator teres, supinator teres, thumb adductor, thumb opponens.
- Recommendations: Use of pillows, swimming, warm scarves, warmth, stretching and elevating.
- Recommended techniques: Spraying and stretching, injections, and PGM release.

4.2.2. Sternocleidomastoid.

- Origin:
  - Sternal fascicle: manubrium of the sternum.
  - Clavicular fascicle: medial third of the clavicle.
- Insertion: Mastoid process and superior occipital curve line (external part).
- Functions:
  - Unilateral: Causes homolateral tilt and contralateral rotation of the head.
  - Bilateral: Performs cervical flexion, although the posterior fibers can generate extension of the cervical spine. It also acts as an accessory muscle in forced breathing, elevating the sternum if the fixed point is on the head.
- Referred pain and PGM:

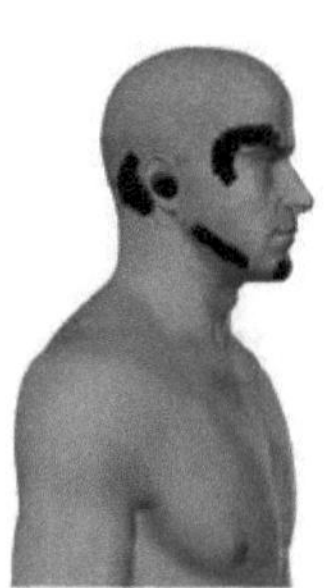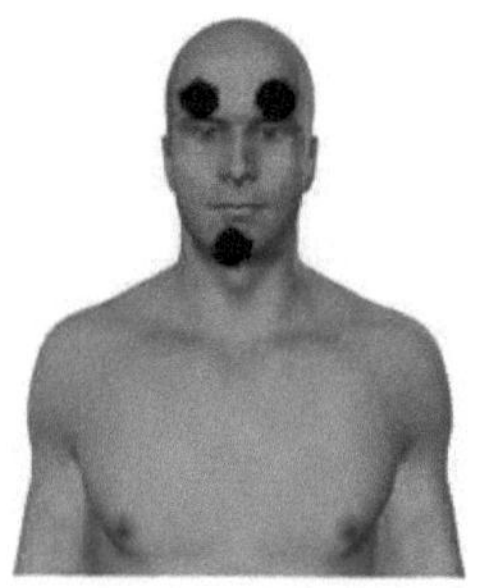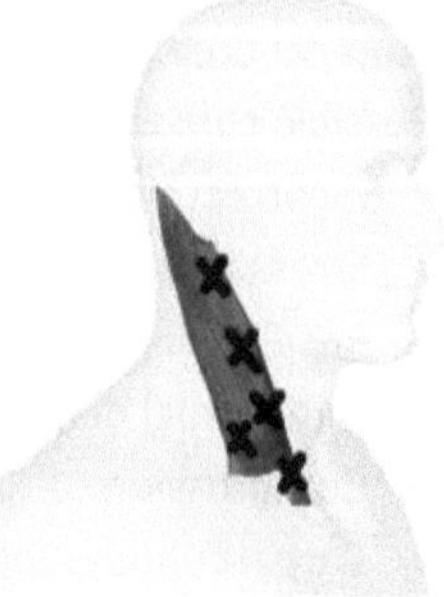

Figure 19. Referred pain represented by black color of the sternocleidomastoid muscle (first and second figure) and PGM represented by black crosses (last figure).

- Symptoms:
  - The sternal fascicle generates referred pain in the mastoid, occiput, supraorbital area and throat.
  - The clavicular fascicle causes pain in the ear and frontal area.
  - In some cases, the muscle may cause dizziness due to rotation of the temporal bone.
- Possible causes:
  - Maintained postures, such as: cervical flexion, flexion with cervical rotation or cervical extension.
  - Paradoxical breathing or chronic respiratory infections.
  - Anxiety and stress.
  - Alterations in other structures, such as the pectoralis major, or even lameness affecting posture.
  - Whiplash or whiplash.
  - Incorrect posture with the head forward.
- Differential diagnosis
  - Otitis.
  - Trigeminal neuralgia.
  - Vestibular dysfunction.
  - Affections in other muscles with similar referred pain: platysma, digastric, splenius, longissimo of the head, semispinal, suboccipital, trapezius, temporal, occipitofrontal, orbicularis oculi, masseter.

4.2.3. Platisma

- Origin: Superficial fascia of the deltoid and pectoral regions.
- Insertion: Mandible, skin of the cheek, angle of the mouth and the orbicularis oris muscle of the lips.
- Actions: Tightens the skin of the neck and lower face. Helps to lower the jaw.

- Referred pain and PGM:

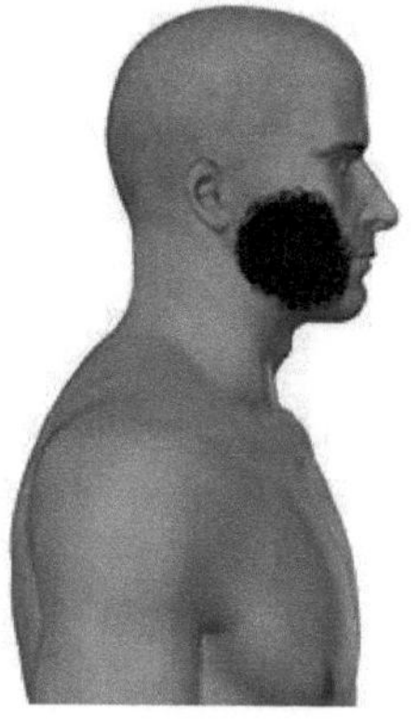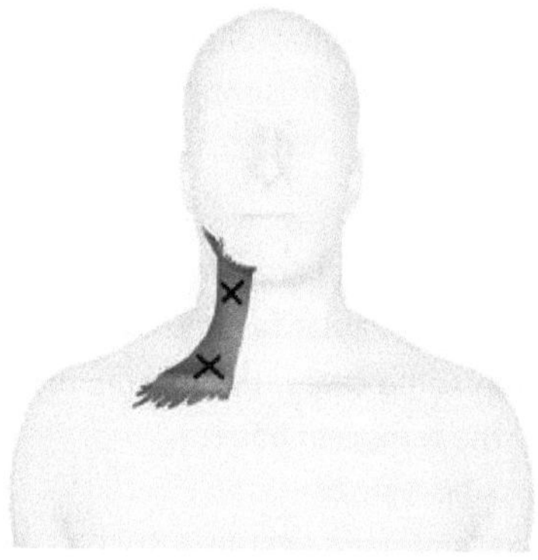

Figure 20. Referred pain represented by black color (first and second figure) and PGMs represented by black crosses (last figure) of the platysma.

- Symptoms: Referred pain in the mandibular area, characterized by a superficial pain with a prickling sensation and paresthesia.
- Possible causes:
  - Temporomandibular joint dysfunction.
  - Keeping the mouth open for prolonged periods of time (such as during dental procedures).
- Differential diagnosis:
  - Dental problems.
  - Trigeminal neuralgia.
- Affection in other muscles with similar referred pain: sternocleidomastoid, temporal, buccinator, masseter, pterygoid.

4.2.4. Suboccipital.

- Major posterior rectus of the head:
  - Origin: Spinous process of C2 (axis).
  - Insertion: Inferior occipital curved line.
- Minor posterior rectus of the head:
  - Origin: Posterior tubercle of C1 (atlas).
  - Insertion: Inferior occipital curved line (covered by the greater rectus).
- Major (or inferior) oblique of the head:
  - Origin: Spinous process of C2 (axis).

- Insertion: Transverse process of C1 (atlas).
- Lesser (or superior) oblique of the head:
    - Origin: Transverse process of C1 (atlas).
    - Insertion: Occipital bone.
- Shares:
    - Neck extension when acting bilaterally.
    - Motor control between the occipital bone, C1 and C2.
    - Posterior rectus abdominis: If contracted unilaterally, it generates homolateral rotation.
    - Oblique major: Performs homolateral tilt and rotation.
    - Lesser oblique: Produces homolateral tilt.
- Referred pain and PGM:

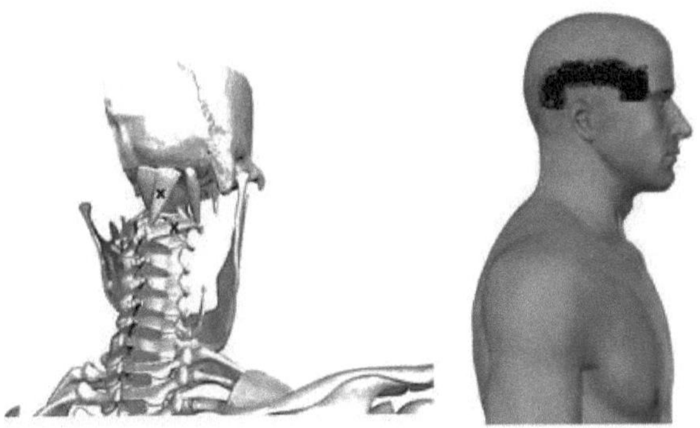

Figure 21. PGMs represented by black crosses (first figure) and referred pain represented in black (second figure) of the suboccipital muscles.

- Symptoms:
    - Tension headache with diffuse pain, difficult to localize.
    - Referred pain over the ears, horizontally, which may reach the eye.
    - Limitation of cervical mobility.
    - Tightness sensation at the base of the occiput, although the patient cannot pinpoint the pain.
- Possible causes:
    - Postures maintained in flexion or extension + rotation.
    - Anteriorized head posture.
    - Direct cold in the area.

- Visual problems or use of bifocal glasses (due to neck movement to improve vision).
- Differential diagnosis:
  - Migraine.
  - Joint dysfunction.
  - Ankylosing spondylitis (due to stiffness and limitation of the neck).
  - Cervical osteoarthritis.
- Alteration of other muscles with similar symptoms: semispinous, longissimus capitis, splenius, sternocleidomastoid, digastric, trapezius, temporalis, occipitofrontalis, masseter.

4.2.5. Multifids

- Origin: It originates in the posterior area of the sacrum, posterosuperior iliac spine, sacroiliac ligaments, mammillary processes of the L1 to L5 vertebrae, transverse processes of T1 to T12 and in the articular processes of the C4 to C7 vertebrae.
- Insertion: It inserts in the spinous processes of the superior vertebrae, sometimes jumping 2 to 4 vertebrae above.
- Functions: When acting bilaterally, they cause extension of the spine. When activated unilaterally, they allow homolateral tilt and contralateral rotation.
- Referred pain and PGM:

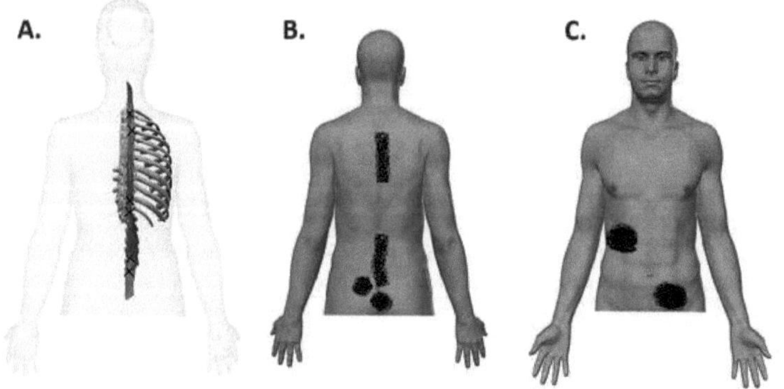

Figure 22. PGMs represented by black crosses (Figure A) and referred pain represented by black color of the multifidus musculature.

- Symptoms: Highly localized pain. Pain radiating to the anterior region, especially in the abdominal area. Posteriorly, the pain manifests in the sacroiliac region and between the scapulae. There may also be hypersensitivity to touch in the coccyx area and restriction of spinal mobility.
- Possible causes:
  - Postures maintained in flexion, inclination or rotation of the trunk.
  - Trauma, such as those resulting from automobile accidents.
  - Dysmetria in the lower extremities.
- Differential diagnosis:
  - Inflammation of the sacroiliac joint (related to diseases such as spondylitis).
  - Coccygodynia.
  - Rib pathologies.
  - Vertebral joint dysfunction.
  - Arthritis and osteoarthritis.
  - Visceral pain.
  - Alterations in other muscles that present similar referred pain, such as rectus abdominis, oblique abdominis, transverse abdominis, trapezius, levator scapulae, infraspinatus, rhomboid, quadratus lumborum, rotator cuff, iliocostalis dorsi, psoas iliacus, gluteus medius, gluteus maximus, piriformis and soleus.
- Recommendations: Posture. Kyphosis due to working position. Number and type of pillows. Work considerations
- Recommended techniques: Spraying and stretching, injections, dry needling and PGM release.

4.2.6. Trunk rotators.

- Origin: Transverse process.
- Insertion: Lamina and transverse or spinous process of the upper vertebrae (usually of the adjacent or second nearest vertebra).
- Actions: Extension of the spine and rotation to the opposite side.

- Referred pain and PGM:

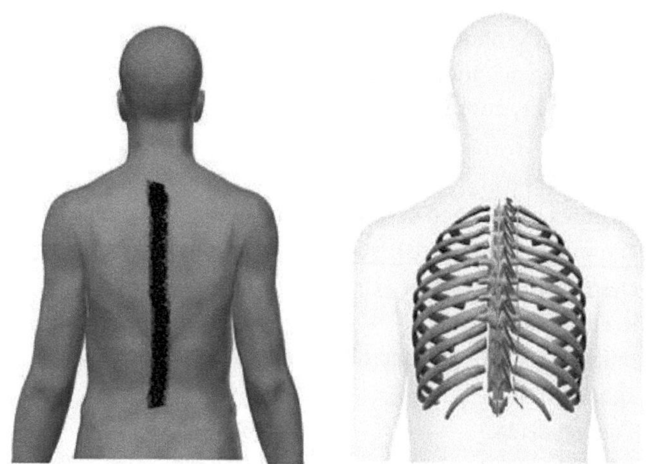

Figure 23. Referred pain depicted in black (left figure) and rotator muscles (right figure).

- Symptoms: Localized pain in the spine, accompanied by hypersensitivity to touch over the spinous processes. The pain may appear with movements of the spine or even present restriction of mobility.
- Possible causes:
  - Maintenance of postures in flexion and/or rotation of the trunk.
  - Trauma such as automobile accidents.
  - Discrepancy in the length of the lower limbs.
- Differential diagnosis:
  - Inflammation of the sacroiliac joint (associated with diseases such as spondylitis).
  - Coccygodynia.
  - Vertebral joint dysfunction.
  - Arthritis and osteoarthritis.
- Alterations in other muscles with similar referred pain: rectus abdominis, trapezius, levator scapulae, rhomboids, quadratus lumborum, multifidus, dorsal iliocostalis, iliac psoas.

4.2.7. Head splenium / neck splenium

- Splenium of the head:
  - Origin: In the posterior cervical ligament and in the spinous processes of the vertebrae from C7 to T3.
  - Insertion: Mastoid process of the temporal bone and in the external portion of the superior curved line of the occipital bone.
- Neck splenium:
  - Origin: Spinous processes of the vertebrae from T3 to T6.
  - Insertion: Transverse processes and posterior tubercles of vertebrae C1 to C3.
- Actions: Both sections, when acting bilaterally, contribute to extension of the cervical spine. If they work unilaterally, they cause tilt and rotation to the same side.
- Referred pain and PGM:

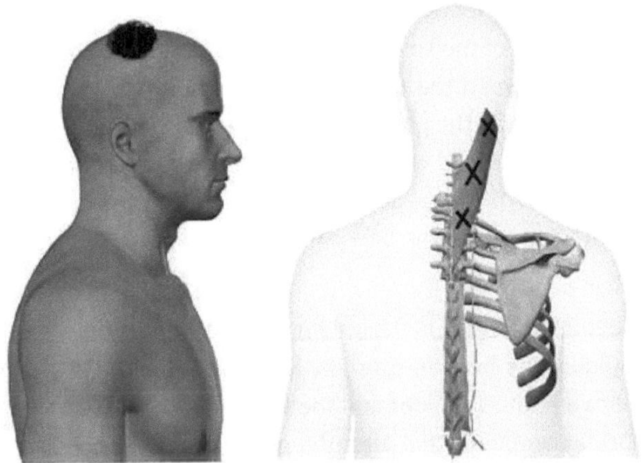

Figure 24. Referred pain depicted in black (left figure) and PGM depicted with black crosses (right figure) of the splenius muscle of the head.

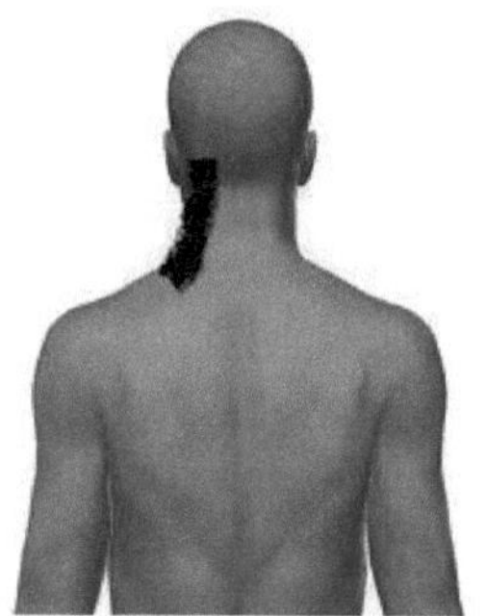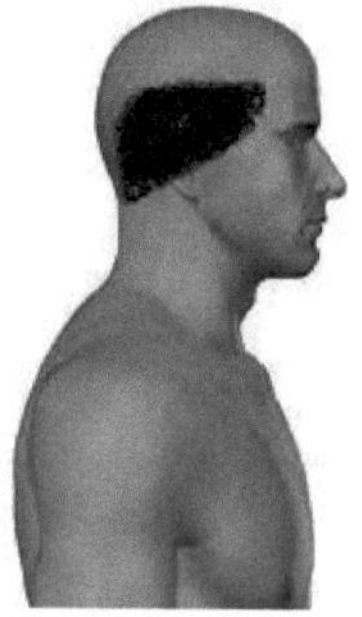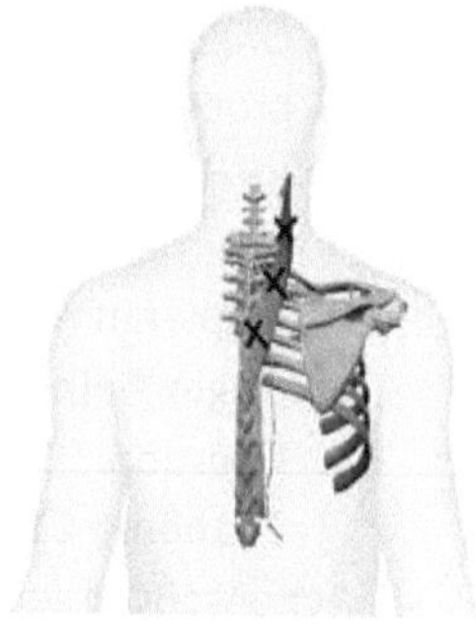

Figure 25. Referred pain represented in black (first and second figure) and PGM represented with black crosses (last figure) of the splenius muscle of the neck.

- Symptoms:

The referred pain of the splenium of the head is located in the upper part of the skull, between the frontal and parietal areas. In the case of the splenius of the neck, the pain radiates to the supraorbital region and part of the temporal area, as well as affecting the upper area of the trapezius muscle. It is one of the muscles that can trigger tension headaches and limit the movements of the cervical spine.

- Possible causes:
  - Keeping the head in flexion for long periods of time.
  - Holding the head in rotation or tilt, as when holding a telephone between the shoulder and the ear.
  - Ocular problems that alter the position of the neck.
  - Whiplash injuries following an automobile accident.
- Differential diagnosis:
  - Migraine headaches.
  - Ocular pathologies (due to referred supraocular pain).
  - Stress.
  - Joint dysfunctions.
  - Conditions in other muscles with similar referred pain: sternocleidomastoid, longissimus head, semispinatus, suboccipital, trapezius, levator scapulae, temporalis, occipitofrontalis.

4.2.8. Very long back.

- Origin: Common sacrolumbar mass.
- Insertion: Transverse processes of the vertebrae up to T1 and proximal ribs.
- Shares:
    - Bilateral: Extends the spine.
    - Unilateral: Tilts the trunk to the same side.
- Referred pain and PGM:

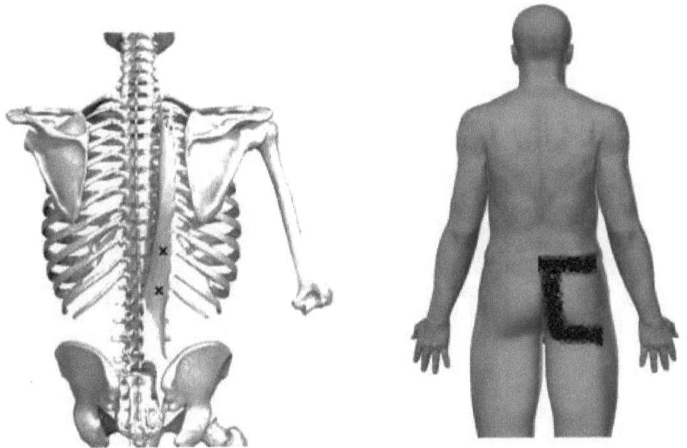

Figure 26. PGM represented with black crosses (first figure) and referred pain represented in black (second figure) of the longissimus dorsi muscle.

- Symptoms: Referred pain in the lower buttock and lumbar area, especially near the iliac. There may be restriction of movement.
- Possible Causes:
    - Postures maintained in flexion and inclination of the trunk.
    - Trauma, such as car accidents.
    - Lower limb dysmetria.
- Differential diagnosis:
    - Inflammation of the sacroiliac joint, as in spondylitis.
    - Coccygodynia.
    - Vertebral joint dysfunction.
    - Arthritis and osteoarthritis.

- Other musculature with similar referred pain: rectus abdominis, latissimus dorsi, quadratus lumborum, iliocostalis lumborum, hamstrings.

4.2.9. Anterior serratus.

- Origin: The serratus anterior muscle originates in the first ten ribs (sometimes only reaching the eighth or ninth rib), with digits inserting into each rib.
- Insertion: Inserted along the medial border of the scapula. The first fingering is attached to the superior angle of the scapula, while the last fingering is attached to the inferior angle.
- Shares:
  - It performs scapula abduction and superior rotation when the ribs act as a fixed point, which facilitates glenohumeral flexion.
  - With the ribs as a fixed point, it displaces the scapula forward (protrusion), preventing the scapula from sliding outward ("flapping").
  - If the fixed point is the scapula, the serratus anterior acts as an inspiratory muscle, lifting the ribs upward.
- Referred pain and PGM:

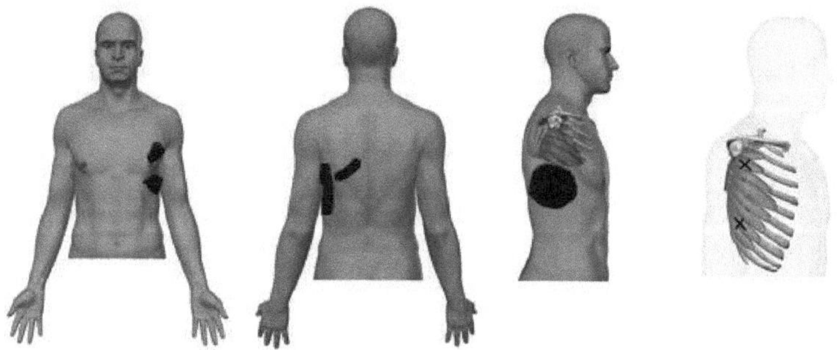

Figure 27. Referred pain represented in black (first, second and third figure) and PGM represented with black crosses (fourth figure) of the serratus anterior muscle.

- Symptoms: The referred pain is located in the medial part of the arm, affecting the last two fingers of the hand, as well as the lower edge of the scapula and along the muscle. Patients often describe a sensation of shortness of breath or shortness of breath, as if something is preventing full respiration. Pain may also occur during inspiration.

- Possible causes:
  - Respiratory diseases such as asthma.
  - Sudden movements (such as a quick twist of the torso at the steering wheel).
  - Intense exercise (due to rapid muscle activation and accelerated breathing).
  - Anxiety and stress.
  - Raise your arms above your head.
- Differential diagnosis:
  - Costochondritis.
  - Problems in the pectoral musculature.
  - Entrapment of the intercostal nerve.
  - Herpes zoster.
  - Rib fractures.
- Affection of other muscles with similar referred pain: subscapularis, pectorals, intercostals, latissimus dorsi, iliocostalis dorsi, triceps brachii, common flexor digitorum, pronator quadratus, little finger abductor, common extensor digitorum.

4.2.10. Posterior serratus

- Superior:
  - Origin: Spinous processes from C7 to T3, posterior cervical ligament and supraspinous ligaments.
  - Insertion: Superior border of the 2nd to 5th ribs.
- Inferior
  - Origin: spinous processes from T11 to L2.
  - Insertion: Inferior border of the 9th to 12th ribs.
- Actions: The upper muscle elevates the ribs, while the lower muscle depresses the ribs. Both aid in respiration, with the upper facilitating inspiration and the lower contributing to expiration.
- Referred pain and PGM:

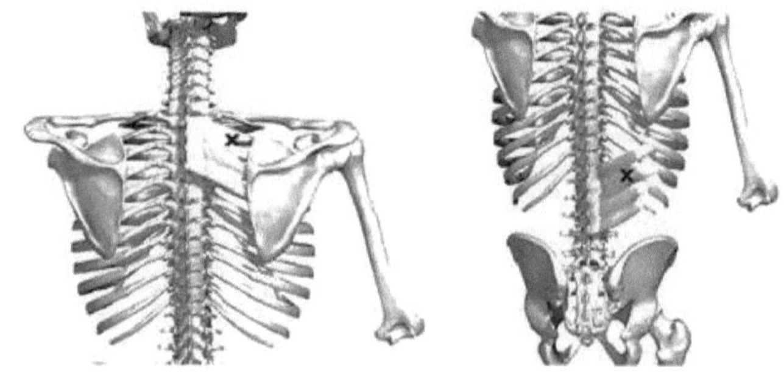

Figure 28. PGM in serratus posterior superior (first figure) and serratus posterior inferior (second figure).

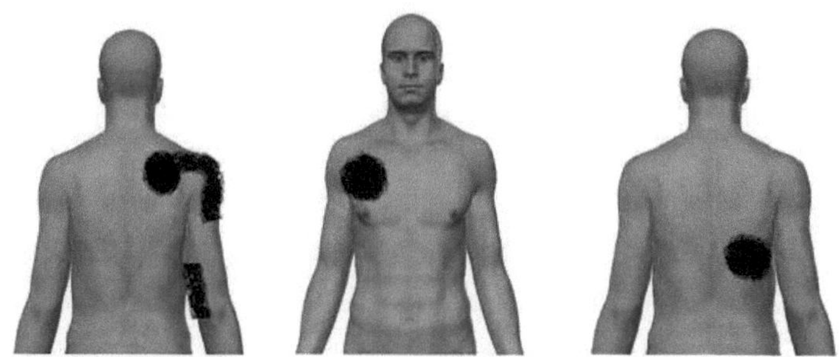

Figure 29. Referred pain for serratus posterior superior (first and second figure) and serratus posterior inferior (last figure).

- Symptoms:
  - The serratus posterior superioris causes referred pain that may extend from the scapula and shoulder to the back of the arm, elbow (epitrochlear area), forearm, wrist and fifth metacarpal. There may also be chest pain. This pain, which is deep and persistent at rest, usually intensifies with weight bearing.
  - The serratus posterioris inferior generates local pain that is usually relieved by stretching.
- Possible causes:
  - Respiratory disorders such as cough or asthma.
  - Anxiety and stress.
  - Scoliosis.
  - Activities with raised arms (e.g., working at high tables).
  - Leg length differences.

- Postures involving trunk rotation.
- Differential diagnosis:
    - Thoracic gorge syndrome.
    - Olecranian bursitis.
    - C7-C8 or C8-T1 radiculopathy.
    - Renal problems.
    - Spinal dysfunction.
- Other muscular alterations with similar pain: scalenes, pectoralis, trapezius, scapula angularis, supraspinatus, rhomboid, teres major, latissimus dorsi, iliocostalis, coracobrachialis, triceps brachii, deltoid, pronator quadratus, little finger abductor.

4.2.11.   Intercostals.

- External intercostals:
    - Origin: Inferior border of the rib (external lip of the costal canal).
    - Insertion: Superior border of the rib immediately below.
    - Arrangement: From dorsal to ventral.
- Internal intercostals:
    - Origin: External lip of the costal canal, at the inferior border of the rib.
    - Insertion: Superior border of the inferior rib.
    - Arrangement: From ventral to dorsal, extending from the mid-axillary line to the edge of the sternum.
- Intimate intercostals:
    - Origin: Internal lip of the costal canal.
    - Insertion: Superior border of the inferior rib.
    - Arrangement: From ventral to dorsal, starting from the posterior rib angle to approximately 6 cm from the sternal border.
- Shares:
    - The external intercostals are inspiratory muscles during respiration, helping to stabilize the rib cage. When contracted on one side, they facilitate contralateral rotation of the thoracic spine.
    - The internal and intimal intercostals act as expiratory muscles and also stabilize the rib cage.
- Referred pain and PGM:

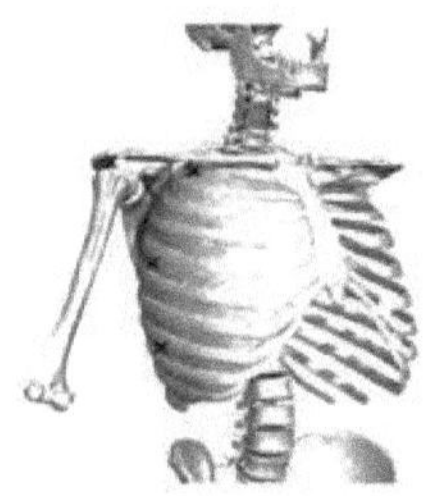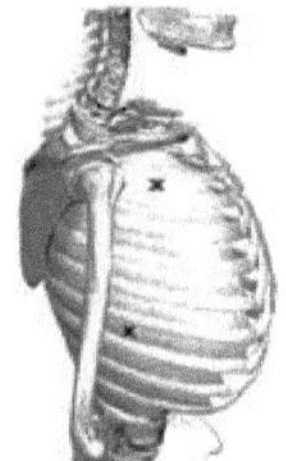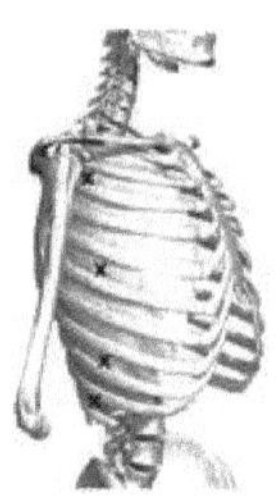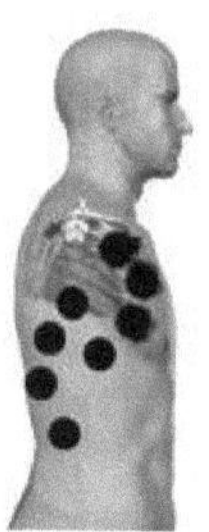

PGMs marked with black crosses of external intercostals (first figure), internal intercostals (second figure) and intimal intercostals (third figure). Referred pain of the intercostal muscles (last figure).

- Symptoms: The referred pain is local and affects the intercostal area. It intensifies with deep breathing, coughing and sneezing. It also generates discomfort on trunk rotation and pain when lifting the arm, due to the limited mobility of the ribs.
- Possible Causes:
  - Thoracic surgery.
  - Trauma such as rib fractures or contusions.
  - Catarrhal processes with coughing and sneezing.
  - Herpes zoster.
  - Postures maintained in trunk rotation or with the arm elevated.
  - Intrathoracic lesions such as pneumothorax.
- Differential Diagnosis
  - Herpes zoster.
  - Rib pathologies.
  - Tietze's syndrome.
  - Intercostal radiculopathy.
- Affection of other muscles with similar referred pain: serratus anterior, diaphragm.

4.2.12.   Broad dorsal.

- Origin: spinous processes from T6 to L5, sacrum (through the thoracolumbar fascia), ribs from 9th to 12th and iliac crest.
- Insertion: Intertubercular groove of the bicipital groove.

- Shares:
  - With the back fixed: Internal rotation, extension and adduction of the shoulder.
  - With both sides working: Trunk extension.
  - With the humerus fixed: Allows movements such as swimming or climbing, and helps in breathing, especially during forced inspiration.
- Referred pain and PGM:

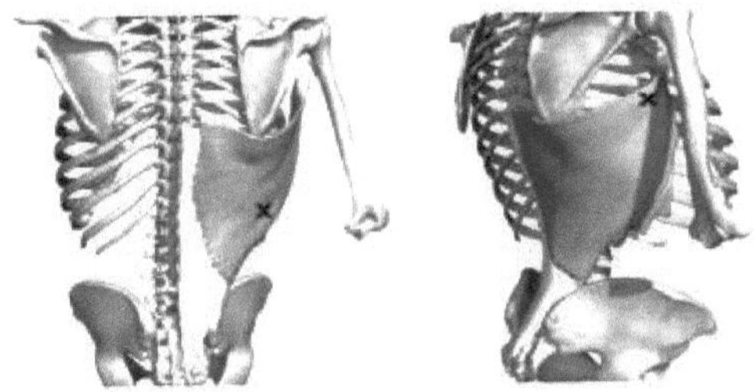

Figure 31. PGM in latissimus dorsi.

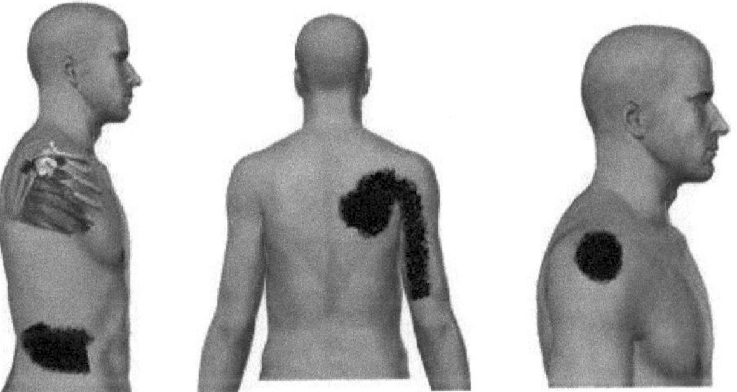

Figure 32. Referred latissimus dorsi pain.

- Symptoms: Referred pain in the angle of the scapula, medial aspect of the arm (similar to radiculopathy), anterior shoulder and over the iliac crest. Pain does not increase with movement or stretching.

- Possible causes:
  - Weight lifting.
  - Repetitive overhead arm activities, such as pull-ups.

- Respiratory disorders.
  - Compressions, such as wearing bras or sleeping on the side.
- Differential Diagnosis:
  - Thoracic pathology, such as cardiopulmonary diseases or rib fractures.
  - C7 radiculopathy.
  - Brachial plexus syndrome.
  - Bicipital tendinopathy.
- Other muscular alterations with similar pain: subscapularis, pectorals, serratus anterior, diaphragm, transverse abdominis, serratus posterior superior, dorsal iliocostalis, dorsal longissimus, anterior brachialis, deltoid, coracobrachialis, biceps brachii.

4.2.13. Square lumbar.

- Origin: Internal lip of the iliac crest and iliolumbar ligament.
- Insertion: Inferior border of the 12th rib and apexes of the transverse processes from L1 to L4.
- Shares:
  - Unilateral: Lateral inclination of the trunk to the same side.
  - Bilateral: Extends the trunk.
  - It fixes the 12th rib, contributing to breathing during inspiration and stabilizes the lumbar spine.
- Referred pain and PGM:

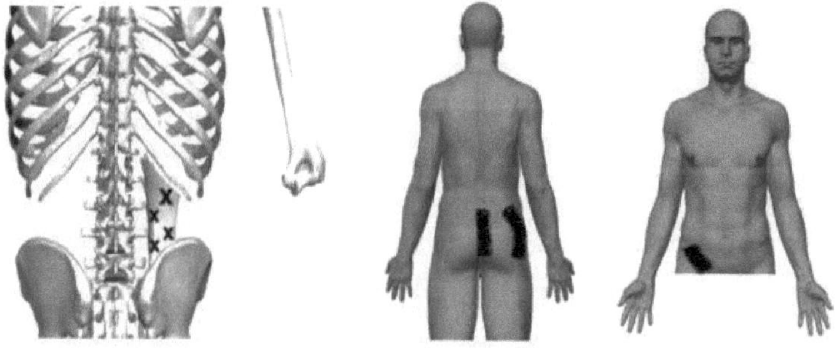

Figure 33. PGMs marked with black crosses of the quadratus lumborum muscle (first figure) Referred pain of the intercostal muscles (second and third figures).

- Symptoms: Referred pain in several areas, including the lower abdomen (up to the groin), the lower gluteal region, the greater trochanter area of the femur and the sacroiliac joint. The pain is deep and there may be hypersensitivity to palpation. Discomfort is aggravated by getting out of bed or a chair, walking with a straight back, prolonged standing or even at rest. Movement increases the pain and there is restriction in flexion and bending of the trunk. Pain may also be experienced when coughing or sneezing.

- Possible causes:
  - Lifting weights in an incorrect posture.
  - Trauma, as in car accidents.
  - Exposure to direct cold.
  - Sudden turns or inclinations of the trunk.
  - Postures maintained in flexion and inclination of the trunk, such as when dressing while standing.
  - Repeated microtrauma, such as in professions involving physical exertion or running on inclined surfaces.
  - Lower limb dysmetria and lameness.
- Differential diagnosis:
  - Trochanteritis and trochanteric bursitis.
  - Herniated disc in the lumbar region.
  - Ciatalgia.
  - Lumbar and sacral joint dysfunction.
  - Inflammation of the sacroiliac joint, which may include spondylitis.
  - Spondylolysis and spondylolisthesis.
  - Costal pathology.
- Other muscles with similar pain: rectus abdominis, oblique abdominis, transverse abdominis, multifidus, rotator cuff, lumbar iliocostalis, longissimus dorsi, psoas iliacus, pectineus, gluteus, piriformis, hamstring, tensor fascia latae, soleus.

4.2.14.   Diaphragm.

- The diaphragm has three groups of fibers:
  - Sternal fibers: Originate from the posterior part of the xiphoid process.
  - Rib fibers: Originate from ribs 7 to 12.

- Lumbar fibers: They originate in the L1 to L3 vertebrae, from the vertebral bodies and the lumbocostal arches (ligaments).
- Insertion: The diaphragm forms the central tendon, which is clover-shaped and lies just below the pericardium. It has no bony insertion and has the appearance of a parachute.
- Actions: It is the main muscle of inspiration. When contracted, the central tendon moves downward and forward, increasing thoracic volume in all dimensions. This occurs when the lower ribs are fixed, allowing more effective air entry into the lungs.
- Referred pain and PGM:

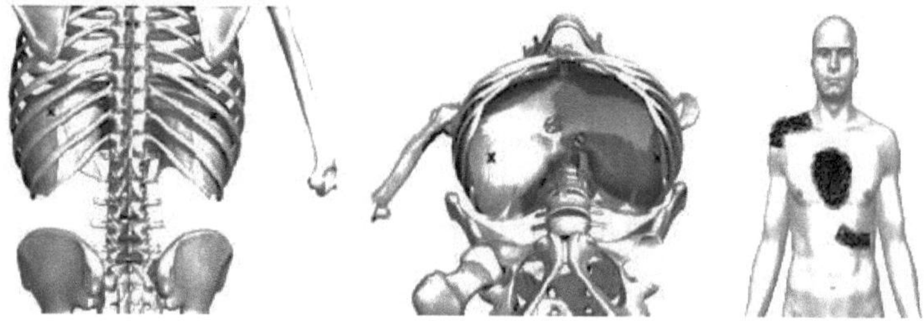

Figure 34. PGMs marked with black crosses of the diaphragm (first and second figure) Referred pain of the diaphragm (third figure).

- Symptoms:
  - Homolateral shoulder pain when the trigger point is in the area of the dome of the diaphragm.
  - Pain in the peripheral costal or precordial area.
  - Lateral costal pinching sensation.
  - Shortness of breath and difficulty breathing deeply.
- Possible causes:
  - Intense exercise requiring rapid or poorly coordinated breathing.
  - Persistent cough or respiratory diseases.
  - Gastric problems due to the anatomical proximity of the diaphragm to the stomach.
- Differential diagnosis:
  - Gastric or hepatic problems (due to the location of the pain).
  - Rib injuries.
  - Respiratory pathologies that cause shortness of breath.
- Alteration of other muscles with similar referred pain: pectoralis, intercostals, subscapularis, oblique abdominis, transverse abdominis,

infraspinatus, latissimus dorsi, biceps brachii, anterior brachialis, coracobrachialis.

4.2.15. Obliques of the abdomen.

- External oblique:
  - Origin: 5th to 12th ribs.
  - Insertion: On the anterior 2/3 of the iliac crest. In the anterior part, it forms an aponeurosis that joins at the linea alba and inserts on the pubis.
- Internal oblique:
  - Origin: In the inguinal ligament and in the anterior 2/3 of the iliac crest (midline), and also in the thoracolumbar fascia.
  - Insertion: 9th to 12th ribs. In addition, it forms an aponeurosis surrounding the rectus abdominis and joins at the linea alba, extending to the costal cartilages of the 7th to 9th and a portion to the pubis.
- Shares:
  - External oblique:
    - Bilaterally: Flexes the trunk, supports the abdominal viscera and facilitates functions such as defecation, urination, delivery and expiration.
    - Unilaterally: Rotates the trunk to the opposite side (contralateral rotation), tilts the trunk to the same side (homolateral tilt) and elevates the pelvis.
  - Internal oblique:
    - Bilaterally: Performs trunk flexion and also assists in defecation, urination, delivery and expiration.
    - Unilaterally: Rotates and tilts the trunk to the same side (homolateral rotation and tilt) and elevates the pelvis.

- Referred pain and PGM:

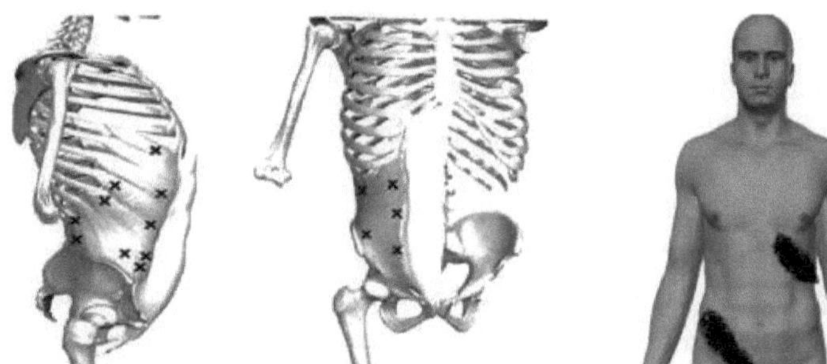

Figure 35. PGMs marked with black crosses (first and second figure) and referred pain (third figure) of the abdominal obliques.

- Symptoms:
    - Myofascial trigger points (MTrPs) in the obliques can cause local pain in several areas:
    - Rib pain.
    - Pain with a feeling of heartburn or pain in the liver area.
    - Lateral and inferior PGMs can cause groin and testicular pain.
    - Alterations in urination due to the involvement of the detrusor muscle of the bladder and sphincter.
    - Limitation or pain in trunk movements, such as bending, flexion and rotation.
    - They can also influence breathing or evacuation problems.
- Possible causes:
    - Childbirth and pregnancy.
    - Respiratory pathology such as colds or cough.
    - Stress and anxiety.
    - Repetitive exercise.
    - Direct trauma.
    - Alterations of the abdominal viscera.
    - Postures maintained for prolonged periods of time.

- Differential diagnosis:
    - Abdominal visceral pathology.
    - Pelvic visceral pathology.
- Alteration of other muscles with similar referred pain, such as the diaphragm, rectus abdominis, transverse abdominis, quadratus

lumborum, multifidus, dorsal iliocostalis, psoas iliacus, pectineus, adductor medius, adductor minimus, and adductor magnus.

4.2.16.   Transversus abdominis.

- Origin:
  - Iliac crest: 2/3 anterior.
  - Inguinal ligament.
  - Ribs 7th to 12th: On the inner sides of the costal cartilages.
  - Thoracolumbar fascia.
- Insertion: It joins the aponeurosis of the internal oblique, to finally insert in the linea alba and pubis.
- Shares:
  - Compresses the abdominal viscera, which helps flatten the abdomen.
  - It facilitates defecation, urination, childbirth, and contributes to expiration during respiration, similar to the obliques.
- Referred pain and PGM:

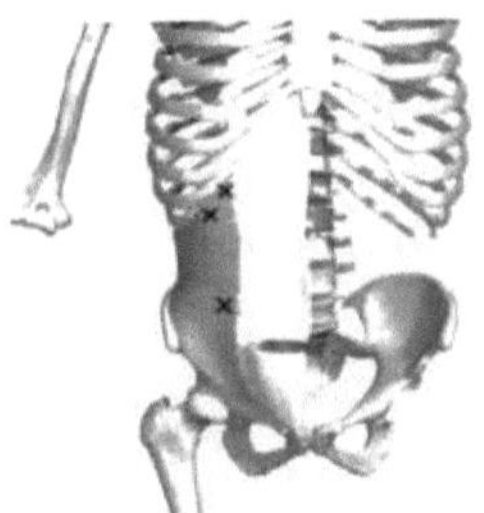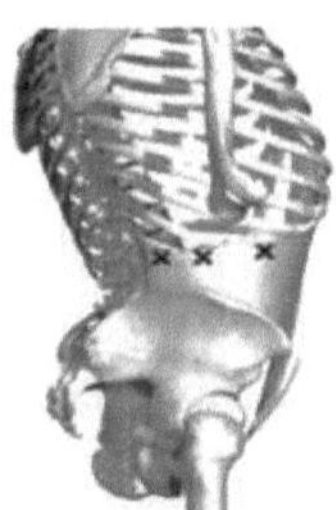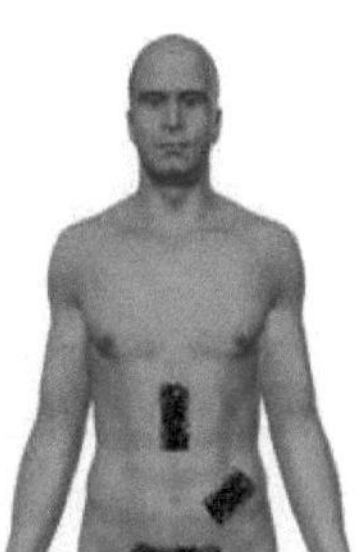

Figure 36. PGMs marked with black crosses (first and second figure) and referred pain (third figure) of the transverse abdominis.

- Symptoms:
  - Referred pain in the pubic area, which can sometimes radiate to the testicles.
  - Referred pain in the iliac crests and anterior abdomen.
  - Sometimes, pain in the area of the xiphoid appendix.
  - Pain sensation similar to costal enthesitis, with discomfort when coughing.
- Possible causes:
  - Catarrhal processes and cough.
  - Visceral pathology.

- Direct trauma.
- Stress and anxiety.
- Differential Diagnosis
  - Abdominal visceral pathology.
  - Pelvic visceral pathology.
  - Costal enthesitis.
- Alteration of other muscles with similar referred pain, such as the diaphragm, rectus abdominis, oblique abdominis, latissimus dorsi, quadratus lumborum, multifidus, dorsal iliocostalis, and pectineus.

4.2.17. Rectus abdominis.

- It originates from two tendons:
  - Lateral tendon: in the pubic spine.
  - Medial tendon: in the symphysis pubis.
- Insertion:
  - The costal cartilages of ribs 5 to 7.
  - The xiphoid process of the sternum.
- Shares:
  - Flexion of the spine by traction of the sternum when the pubis is the fixed point.
  - It contributes to expiration by pulling the ribs downward.
  - If the ribs are the fixed point, it elevates the pelvis, decreasing lumbar lordosis and contributes to pelvic stabilization.
- Referred pain and PGM:

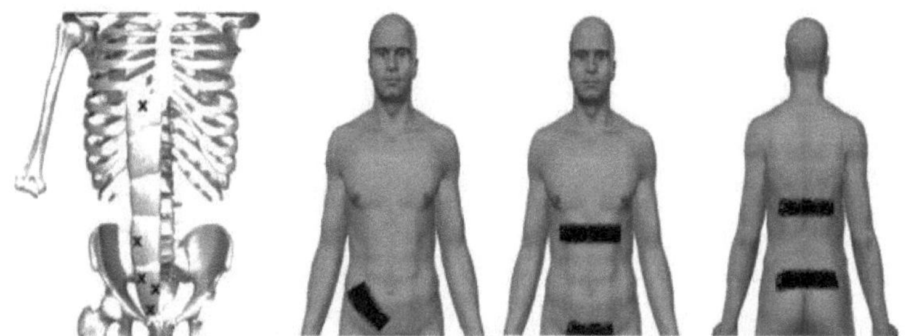

Figure 37. PGMs marked with black crosses (first figure) and referred abdominal pain (second, third and fourth figures) of the rectus abdominis.

- Symptoms:

- In PGMs of the upper fibers, the pain refers to the mid-back and gastric region and may cause digestive discomfort.
- More lateral PGMs cause referred pain in the area of the iliac spines (on the right side, pain may be felt near the appendix).
- Lower PGMs cause pain in the lower back (including sacrum, iliacs and upper buttocks) and pubic region, which can cause dysmenorrhea.
- Possible causes:
  - Gastric alterations (such as ulcer).
  - Scars from surgery.
  - Direct trauma.
  - Intense or forced exercise.
  - Persistent cough.
  - Emotional tension.
  - Prolonged postures in flexion of the trunk.
- Differential diagnosis:
  - Visceral pathology (appendicitis, liver disorders, hiatal hernia).
  - Pelvic viscera pathology (bladder, ovaries).
  - Gynecologic pathology.
- Alteration of other muscles with similar referred pain: oblique abdominis, transverse abdominis, serratus posterior inferior, quadratus lumborum, quadratus lumborum, multifidus, rotator cuff, iliocostalis, longissimus dorsi, psoas iliacus, pectineus, adductor medius, adductor minimus, adductor magnus.

4.2.18. Square lumbar.

- Origin: Internal lip of the iliac crest and iliolumbar ligament.
- Insertion: Inferior border of the 12th rib and apexes of the transverse processes of the vertebrae L1 to L4.
- Shares:
  - Acting unilaterally, it causes homolateral trunk tilt.
  - If acting bilaterally, it contributes to trunk extension.
  - Fixes the 12th rib, which helps during inspiration.
  - Stabilizes the lumbar spine.
- Referred pain and PGM:

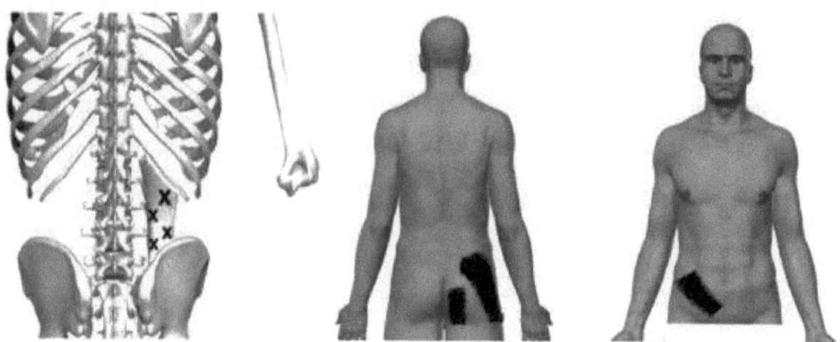

Figure 38. PGMs marked with black crosses (first figure) and referred pain (second and third figures) of the quadratus lumborum.

- Symptoms:
    - Lumbar square generates referred pain in several areas, such as: the lower abdomen (which may extend to the groin), the lower part of the buttock, the area around the greater trochanter of the femur, and the sacroiliac joint. The pain is deep, and sometimes there is hypersensitivity in the area on palpation.
    - Discomfort is reported when getting out of bed or out of a chair, walking with the back upright or standing for long periods of time, even at rest. Movements aggravate the pain considerably. There is limitation in flexion and bending of the trunk. Pain is also experienced when coughing or sneezing, as the muscle stabilizes the 12th rib.
- Possible causes:
    - Lifting heavy objects with bad posture.
    - Trauma, as in a car accident.
    - Direct exposure to cold in the area.
    - Sudden movements of rotation or inclination of the trunk.
    - Maintaining postures in flexion or inclination of the trunk for long periods of time (e.g., dressing while standing).
    - Repeated microtrauma (in professions such as gardeners or cleaners, or when running on inclined surfaces).
    - Differences in the length of the lower limbs or lameness.
- Differential diagnosis:
    - Trochanteritis or trochanteric bursitis.
    - Herniated disc in the lumbar region of the spine.
    - Ciatalgia.

- Joint dysfunction in the lumbar or sacral spine.
  - Inflammation of the sacroiliac joint (including conditions such as spondylitis).
  - Spondylolysis and spondylolisthesis.
  - Rib pathologies.
- Muscle alterations with similar referred pain: rectus abdominis, oblique abdominis, transverse abdominis, multifidus, rotators, lumbar iliocostalis, dorsalis longus, psoas iliacus, pectineus, gluteus, piriformis, hamstring, tensor fascia latae, soleus.

4.3. Shoulder and arm muscles.

4.3.1. Trapeze.

- Origin:
  - Superior: Superior occipital curve line and external occipital protuberance. Posterior nuchal ligament. Spinous processes of the C7 vertebra.
  - Middle: spinous processes of the vertebrae T1 to T5, and supraspinous ligaments.
  - Inferior: spinous processes of the vertebrae T6 to T12, and supraspinous ligaments.

- Insertion:
  - Superior: Lateral third of the clavicle.
  - Middle: Upper surface of the spine of the scapula and acromion.
  - Lower: Scapula (tubercle at the medial end of the spine).
- Shares:
  - If the fixed point is the upper extremity: When acting bilaterally, they produce neck extension. Unilaterally, they cause contralateral rotation and homolateral inclination of the neck, actions performed mainly by the upper fibers of the trapezius.
  - If the fixed point is the spine: Stabilizes the scapula during arm movements. The upper and lower fibers contribute to the rotation of the scapula (moving the glenoid upward). The superior fibers elevate the scapula together with the angular muscle, while the medial fibers collaborate with the superior and inferior fibers in scapular rotation.
- Referred pain and PGM:

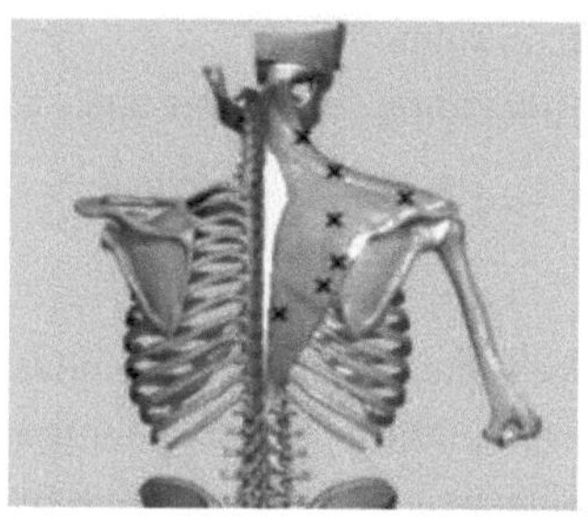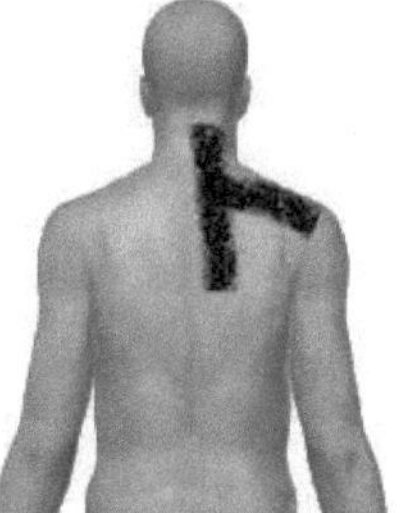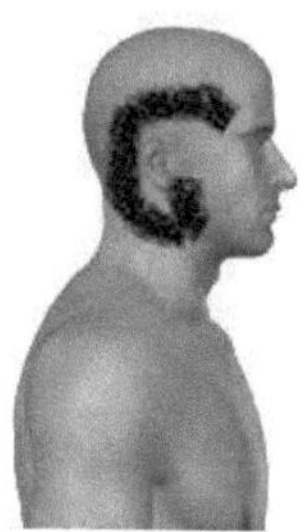

Figure 39. PGMs marked with black crosses (first figure) and referred pain (second and third figures) of the trapezius muscle.

A myofascial trigger point (MTrP) is located in the angle formed by the trapezius, at the base of the cervical spine, and another in the direction of the shoulder, on the spine of the scapula. It is also possible to find more points in the medial region of the medial border of the scapula. It is necessary to differentiate them from other muscles present in the area, such as the ileocostal or rhomboids.

- Symptoms:
  - The trapezius is one of the muscles that contribute to tension headache. The presence of several TMPs can generate pain in different areas. Radiating pain mainly affects the nape of the neck, behind the ear, the forehead and sometimes the angle of the jaw. Other trigger points radiate pain to the back of the shoulder, over the spine of the scapula, as well as to the base of the head, the nape of the neck, the dorsal region of the back and the distal third of the spine of the scapula. PGMs near the spinous processes cause more localized pain, and others at the medial border of the scapula.
  - Patients often report limited mobility of the cervical spine, accompanied by neck stiffness. Some also experience discomfort due to the weight of coats, bags or backpacks, which can cause pain in the shoulders and scapula. In certain cases, patients describe a shivering or goose bumps sensation in the arm along its lateral aspect, linked to the PGMs of the trapezius.
- Possible causes:
  - Cervical sprain or "whiplash" (whiplash).
  - Altered body posture with elevated shoulders.

- Repetitive movements or postures maintained with arms raised above the head.
  - Compression from heavy clothing, coats, bags or backpacks.
  - Prolonged postures with the head in flexion or extension.
- Differential diagnosis:
  - Migraine headaches.
  - Neuralgias.
  - Joint dysfunction.
  - Ankylosing spondylitis, due to cervical stiffness and limitation.
  - Arthrosis.
- Involvement of other muscles that may cause similar referred pain: scalenes, sternocleidomastoid, digastric, splenius, longissimus capitis, semispinatus, suboccipitalis, angularis scapulae, supraspinatus, infraspinatus, rhomboid, teres major, serratus posterior superior, multifidus, rotator cuff, dorsal iliocostalis, temporalis, occipitofrontalis, deltoid.

4.3.2. Angular of the scapula.

- Origin: Transverse processes of the C1 to C4 vertebrae.
- Insertion: Superior angle of the scapula, between the superior angle and the spine of the scapula.
- Shares:
  - If the fixed point is the scapula:
    - Bilaterally: Perform neck extension.
    - Unilaterally: Performs homolateral tilt and homolateral rotation of the neck.
  - If the fixed point is the cervical vertebrae: Elevate the scapula and make a depression of the glenoid cavity.
- Referred pain and PGM:
  - One is located in the middle of the muscular belly.
  - Another is located near the spine of the scapula, in its medial area.

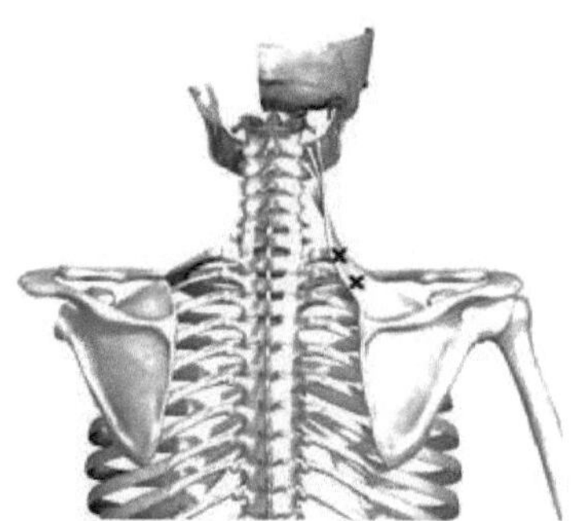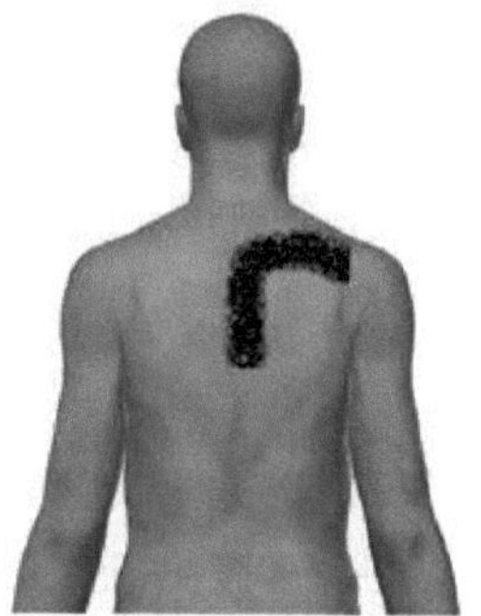

Figure 40. PGMs marked with black crosses (first figure) and referred pain (second figure) of the angularis scapulae muscle.

- Symptoms:
  - Pain referred to the neck, internal border of the scapula, and posterior shoulder area.
  - Stiffness and difficulty in moving the neck, especially in rotation, as it will be limited on both sides due to pain when contracting and stretching the muscle.
- Possible causes:
  - Postures maintained in scapula elevation, such as holding the phone between shoulder and ear or use of canes and crutches.
  - Anxiety and stress.
  - Direct cold on the area.
  - Maintained pressure, such as carrying backpacks or bags.
  - Poor sleeping posture, such as using a pillow that is too low when sleeping on the side.
- Differential diagnosis:
  - Joint dysfunction or winged scapula.
  - Neurological entrapment.
  - Ankylosing spondylitis (due to stiffness).
  - Arthrosis.
- Alteration of other muscles with similar referred pain: scalenes, splenius, trapezius, supraspinatus, infraspinatus, rhomboid, serratus posterior superior, multifidus, rotator cuff, deltoid, triceps brachii.

    4.3.3. Rhomboids (major and minor).

- Major:

- Origin: Spinous processes of the T2 to T5 vertebrae and supraspinous ligament.
  - Insertion: Internal border of the scapula.
- Minor:
  - Origin: Spinous processes of the C7 and T1 vertebrae, and common posterior cervical ligament.
  - Insertion: Internal border of the scapula.
- Actions: Both muscles bring the scapulae closer together. Since the fibers are oblique, they also cause an internal tilt of the scapula, moving the glenoid downward.
- Referred pain and PGM:

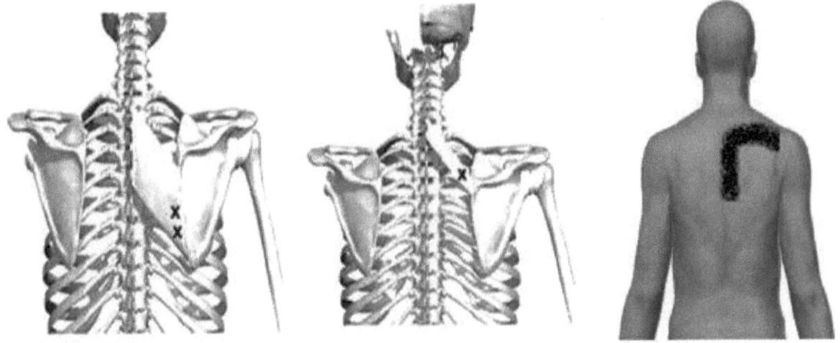

Figure 41. PGMs of the greater rhomboid muscle (first figure) marked with black crosses and lesser rhomboid (second figure) and referred pain (third figure).

- Symptoms: The referred pain is localized at the inner border of the scapula. Some patients report crunching or crackling when moving the arm.
- Possible causes:
  - Maintain postures in flexion and abduction of the arm (as when painting a wall).
  - Prolonged postures with the shoulders in internal rotation (such as when studying, sewing, etc.).
  - Scoliosis.
  - Thoracic surgeries.
- Differential diagnosis: Joint dysfunction between the scapula and the shoulder.

- Affection of other muscles with similar referred pain: scalenes, trapezius, levator scapulae, infraspinatus, serratus posterior superior, multifidus, rotator cuff, iliocostalis dorsi.

4.3.4. Pectoralis minor.

- Origin: Ribs 3 to 5, near the costal cartilages, with a part in the aponeurosis and intercostal muscles.
- Insertion: Coracoid process of the scapula, extending also to the medial border and superior surface of the scapula.
- Shares:
  - If the ribs are the fixed point, perform an antepulsion of the shoulder (also lowering it), pulling the coracoid process downward and rotating the scapula, separating the inferior angle and moving it away from the ribs.
  - If the coracoid process is the fixed point, it acts as an inspiratory muscle during forced breathing.
- Referred pain and PGM:

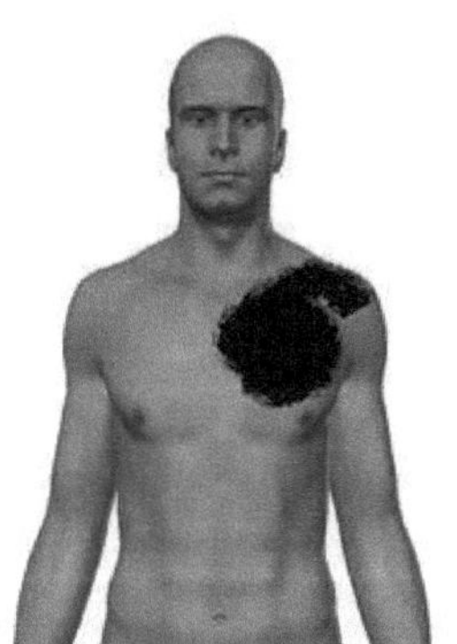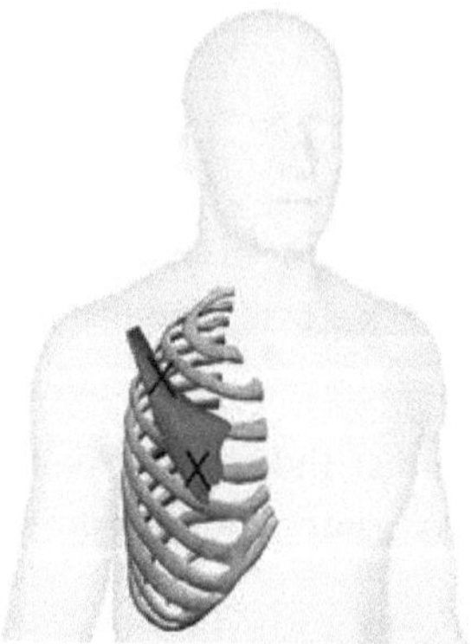

Figure 42. Referred pain represented in black (first figure) and PGM represented with black crosses (second figure) of the pectoralis minor muscle.

- Symptoms:
  - Referred pain in the shoulder, chest (precordial area) and inner arm. There may also be referred pain in the mammary region (telalgia).

- There is a possibility of compression of the brachial plexus or even vascular structures, which may cause restrictions in arm movements or difficulty in performing them.
- Possible causes:
  - Whiplash (whiplash).
  - Problems in the respiratory system.
  - Direct trauma to the area.
  - Compressions in the area (such as those caused by a backpack or clothing straps).
- Differential diagnosis:
  - Thoracic gorge syndrome.
  - Biceps tendinopathy (many patients are misdiagnosed with this condition).
  - Vascular problems.
- Affection of other muscles with similar referred pain: scalenes, subscapularis, pectoralis major, infraspinatus, serratus anterior, diaphragm, serratus posterior superior, latissimus dorsi, coracobrachialis, deltoid, biceps brachii, common extensor digitorum, triceps brachii, common flexor digitorum, pronator quadratus, little finger abductor, brachialis anterior.

4.3.5. Pectoralis major

- Origin:
  - Clavicular portion: It originates in the middle third of the anterior border of the clavicle.
  - Sternal portion: It is located in the front part of the sternum, approximately up to the height of the sixth and seventh costal cartilage. It also inserts on the costal cartilages and on the aponeurosis of the oblique muscle of the abdomen.
- Insertion: The pectoralis major inserts into the outer lip of the bicipital groove of the humerus, with a tendon that divides into two parts: one deep and one more superficial.
- Shares:
  - Performs adduction and internal rotation of the glenohumeral joint, with the sternum as a fixed point.
  - With the arms fixed, both pectorals act as inspiratory muscles during forced breathing.

- The clavicular portion also participates in the flexion of the glenohumeral joint, while the sternal portion performs the extension of the glenohumeral joint and, during the climbing action, tracts the trunk forward and upward.
- Referred pain and PGM:

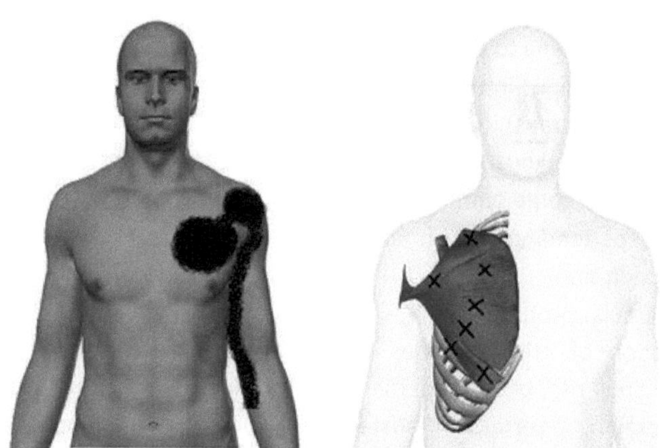

Figure 43. Referred pain represented in black (first figure) and PGM represented with black crosses (second figure) of the pectoralis major muscle.

- Symptoms:
  - Although the pectoralis minor usually generates more clinical, trigger points of the pectoralis major can refer pain from the clavicular portion towards the shoulder, while the sternal portion can generate referred pain in the chest, precordial area and even in the medial region of the forearm and the last three fingers, which can be confused with myocardial infarction pain. The most lateral points may cause pain in the nipple region, causing hypersensitivity.
  - These trigger points also restrict abduction and extension of the glenohumeral joint, and may affect neighboring muscles such as the sternocleidomastoid due to its insertion on the clavicle.
- Possible causes:
  - Overloads (frequent in gym activities).
  - Prolonged posture with shoulders in internal rotation (as when studying with elbows resting).

- Anxiety, since the pectoralis major is an accessory muscle in respiration.
  - After a heart attack, due to pain in areas of the muscle that can activate trigger points.
- Differential diagnosis:
  - Myocardial infarction.
  - Tendinopathy of the biceps brachii, due to pain in the area of the bicipital tendon of the clavicular portion.
  - C7-C8 radiculopathy or brachial plexus syndrome.
  - Respiratory problems in the thoracic region.
  - Tietze's syndrome.
  - Epitroclealgia.
- Affection of other muscles with similar referred pain: Deltoid, scalenes, subscapularis, subclavian, pectoralis minor, serratus anterior, diaphragm, infraspinatus, posterior superior serratus, latissimus dorsi, biceps brachii, triceps brachii, common flexor digitorum, pronator quadratus, little finger abductor, coracobrachialis, common extensor digitorum.

4.3.6. Deltoid

- Origin:
  - Anterior fibers: Anterior border of the lateral portion of the clavicle.
  - Middle fibers: Acromion of the scapula.
  - Posterior fibers: Spine of the scapula.
- Insertion: The three portions of the deltoid muscle insert into the deltoid tuberosity of the humerus.
- Shares:
  - Primarily, the deltoid performs shoulder abduction, with the medial fibers being the most active in this movement.
  - The anterior and posterior fibers stabilize the humeral head during abduction.
  - The anterior fibers also contribute to flexion and internal rotation of the shoulder, while the posterior fibers are responsible for extension and external rotation.

- If the shoulder is at 90º of abduction, the anterior fibers act as adductors anteriorly, and the posterior fibers act as adductors posteriorly.
- Referred pain and PGM:

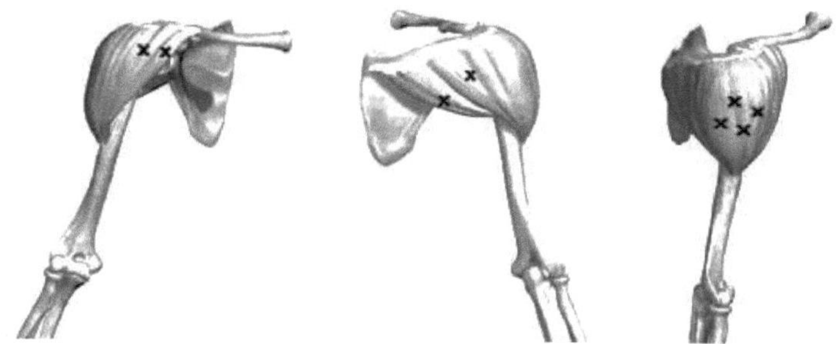

Figure 44. PGM depicted with black crosses of the anterior fibers (first figure), posterior fibers (second figure), and middle fibers (third figure) of the deltoid muscle.

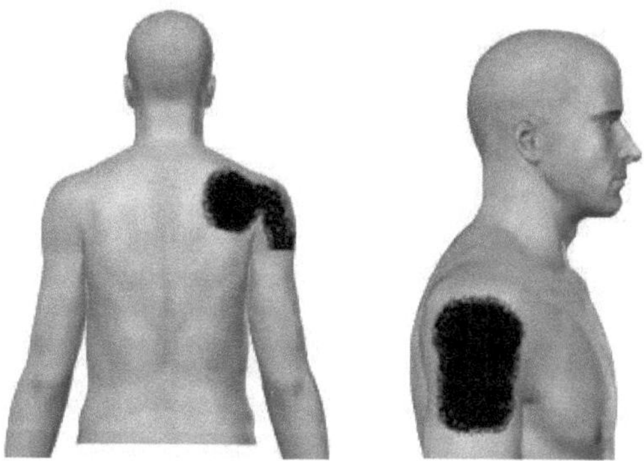

Figure 45. Referred pain depicted in black of the deltoid muscle.

- Symptoms:
  - The referred pain is usually located in the lateral and posterior part of the shoulder, and sometimes it can radiate towards the anterior area. It may also occur in the arm, although it does not usually reach the elbow, being concentrated in the muscle belly. In some cases, there may be pain at rest.
  - There is a marked limitation in shoulder mobility, and pain increases with movement. Patients may report difficulty abducting

the shoulder or performing everyday tasks, such as bringing a fork
to the mouth.
- Possible causes:
  - Rear area:
    - Intramuscular injections.
    - Excessive exercise, such as skiing.
    - Direct trauma.
  - Middle zone:
    - Repetitive movements in abduction.
    - Postures maintained with the shoulder in adduction.
    - Direct trauma.
  - Previous zone:
    - Direct trauma.
    - To hold on to something to prevent a fall.
    - Repetitive movements with the arms above shoulder level (such
      as painting a wall).

- Differential diagnosis:
  - Radiculopathy in nerve roots C5-C6, C6-C7.
  - Subacromial or subdeltoid bursitis.
  - Arthritis.
- Joint dysfunction: involvement of other muscles with similar referred
  pain: subscapularis, pectorals, diaphragm, trapezius, levator scapulae,
  supraspinatus, infraspinatus, teres, serratus posterior, latissimus
  dorsi, iliocostalis dorsi, anterior brachialis, coracobrachialis, biceps
  brachii, triceps brachii.

4.3.7. Supraspinatus.

- Origin: Supraspinous fossa of the scapula.
- Insertion: Superior cartilage of the trochlea of the humerus.
- Shares:
  - Together with the rest of the rotator cuff muscles, it holds the
    humeral head in the glenoid fossa.
  - Perform shoulder abduction in the first few degrees
    (approximately the first 15°).
- Referred pain and PGM:

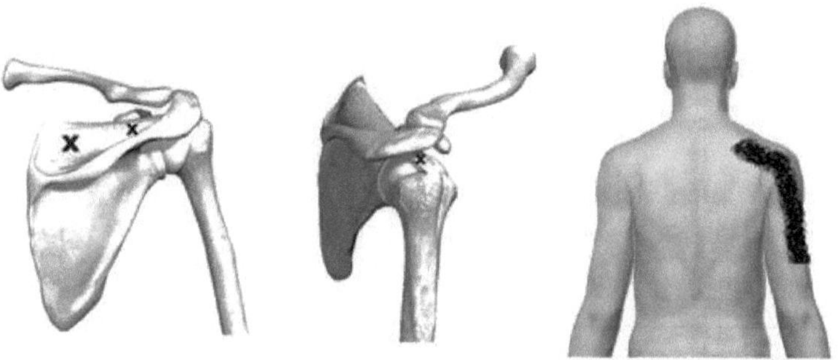

Figure 46. PGM depicted with black crosses (first and second figure) and referred pain depicted in black (third figure) of the supraspinatus.

- Symptoms:
  - Referred pain in the lateral aspect of the arm and shoulder, sometimes reaching the epicondyle.
  - Pain at night and at rest.
  - Difficulty raising the arm above the shoulder (affecting activities such as reaching for objects, combing hair, or brushing teeth).
  - Limitation of shoulder abduction.
- Possible causes:
  - Repetitive work or prolonged postures with the arms above the shoulder (for example, when performing barbell pull-ups).
  - Carrying weight with arms in slight shoulder abduction (as when carrying shopping bags with arms slightly apart).
  - Differential diagnosis
  - Deltoid or subacromial bursitis.
  - Radiculopathy of C5-C6.
  - Capsulitis.
  - Tendinopathy of the shoulder musculature.
  - Epicondylalgia.
- Referred pain due to alteration of other muscles such as: Scalenes, subclavian, trapezius, angularis scapulae, teres major, serratus posterior superior, triceps brachii, deltoid, anconeus, brachioradialis, and common extensor digitorum.

  4.3.8. Infraspinatus.

- Origin: infraspinous fossa of the scapula.

- Insertion: Medial cartilage of the trochlea of the humerus.
- Shares:
  - Together with the rest of the rotator cuff muscles, it helps to maintain the humeral head in the glenoid cavity.
  - Performs external rotation of the shoulder.
- Referred pain and PGM:

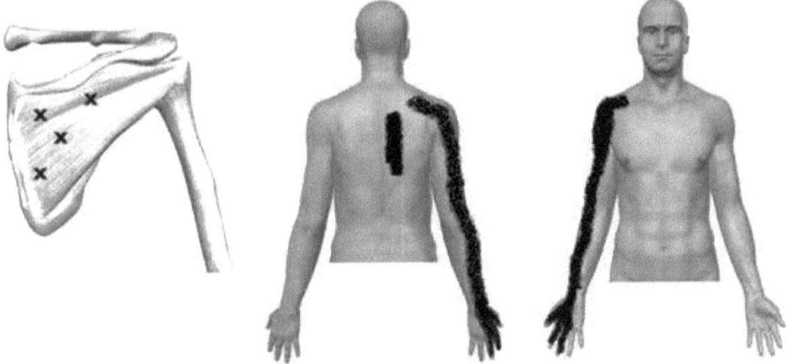

Figure 47. PGM depicted with black crosses (first figure) and referred pain depicted in black (second and third figures) of the infraspinatus.

- Symptoms:
  - Referred pain in the anterior aspect of the shoulder, extending towards the muscle belly area of the biceps brachii and, occasionally, towards the forearm and the first three fingers.
  - More proximal trigger points may generate pain at the medial border of the scapula.
  - Night pain and discomfort when attempting to flex the shoulder above the head or when moving it backwards (difficulty reported by women when fastening their bra).
- Possible causes:
  - Postures maintained with the arm elevated or in extension.
  - Direct trauma with the shoulder in internal rotation (e.g., falling and holding on to a railing or leaning on skis to avoid a fall).
- Differential diagnosis:
  - Tendinopathy of the biceps brachii.
  - Frozen shoulder.
  - Radiculopathy of C5-C6.
  - Arthritis.

- Referred pain due to alteration of other muscles such as: Scalenes, subscapularis, subclavian, pectorals, diaphragm, trapezius, angularis scapulae, rhomboids, latissimus dorsi, multifidus, rotators, iliocostalis dorsi, brachialis anterior, biceps brachii, coracobrachialis, deltoid, and index extensor.

4.3.9. Minor round.

- Origin: Lateral border of the scapula (dorsal surface).
- Insertion: Trochlea of the humerus, diaphysis of the humerus, and capsule of the glenoid joint.
- Actions: Collaborates with the rotator cuff muscles to maintain the head of the humerus in the glenoid cavity. Facilitates external rotation of the shoulder and slight adduction of the shoulder.
- Referred pain and PGM:

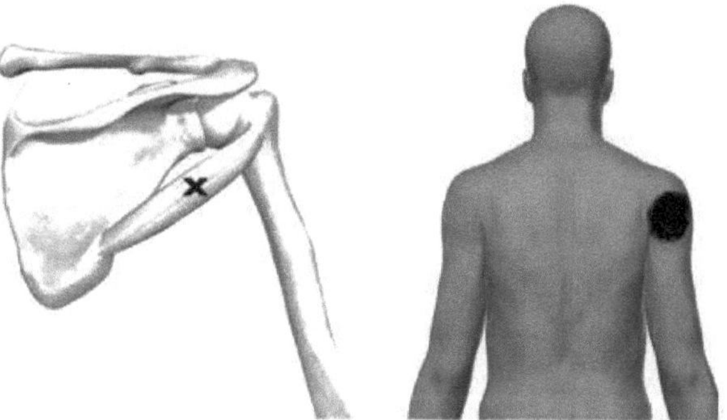

Figure 48. PGM depicted with black crosses (first figure) and referred pain depicted in black (second figure) of the teres minor muscle.

- Symptoms: radiating pain in the lateral part of the arm, near the deltoid and under the head of the humerus, in the form of a cuff. Although it does not restrict movement, the pain increases when attempting to raise or bring the arm backwards.
- Possible Causes:
  - Direct trauma with the shoulder in internal rotation (e.g., falling and holding on to a railing, or skiing with strong support on skis).
  - Automobile accidents while holding the steering wheel.
  - Postures held with the arm raised or extended backwards (as in volleyball).

- Differential Diagnosis:
  - Deltoid bursitis.
  - Joint dysfunction.
  - Other muscular alterations with similar pain: Deltoid.

4.3.10.   Larger round.

- Origin: Dorsal aspect of the inferior angle of the scapula.
- Insertion: Lesser lip of the bicipital slide on the humerus.
- Actions: Facilitates shoulder extension from a flexed position, adduction and internal rotation.
- Referred pain and PGM:

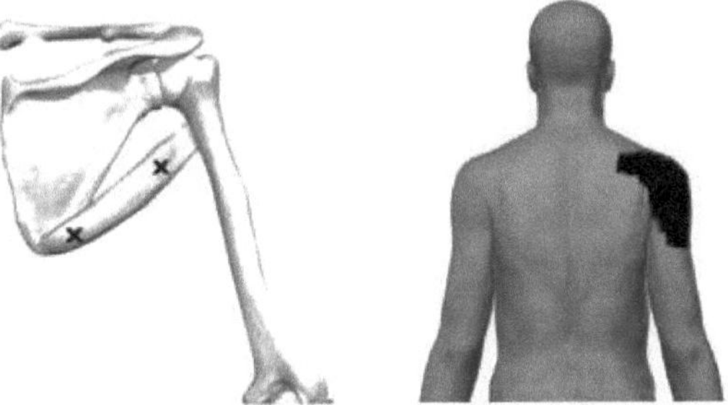

Figure 49. PGM represented with black crosses (first figure) and referred pain represented in black (second figure) of the teres major muscle.

- Symptoms: Deep pain in the posterior shoulder area near the deltoid. Patients may experience hyperalgesia, with pain that increases with minimal stimuli and may be persistent at rest. Pain intensifies when the arm is raised above the head.
- Possible causes:
  - Activities or postures that resist internal rotation of the shoulder.
  - Postures or activities maintained with the arm elevated above shoulder level.
- Differential diagnosis:
  - Subacromial or deltoid bursitis.
  - Brachial plexus syndrome or thoracic gorge syndrome.
  - Calcifications in the supraspinatus tendon.
  - Radiculopathy of C5-C6 or C6-C7.

- Other muscular alterations with similar pain: trapezius, scapula angularis, supraspinatus, serratus posterior superior, iliocostalis dorsi, triceps brachii, deltoid.

4.3.11.　Subscapularis.

- Origin: Scapular fossa. Also in the fascia that separates this muscle from the teres major and the long portion of the triceps brachii.
- Insertion: Trochlea of the humerus and the anterior part of the glenohumeral joint capsule.
- Shares:
  - Internal rotation of the shoulder.
  - It contributes to the stabilization of the glenohumeral joint, keeping the head of the humerus in the glenoid cavity.
- Referred pain and PGM:

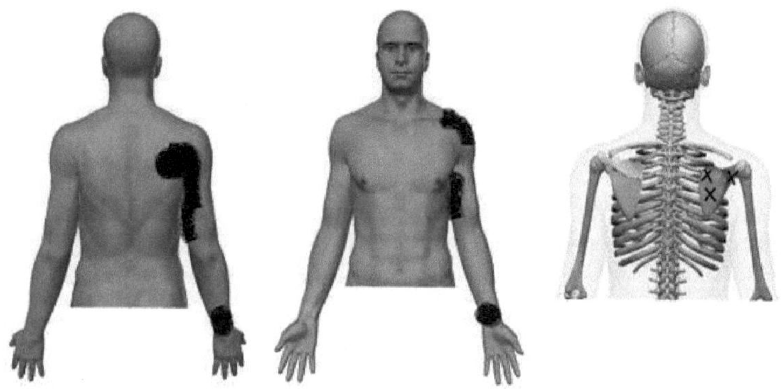

Referred pain represented in black (first and second figure) and PGM represented with black crosses (last figure) of the subscapularis muscle.

- Symptoms:
  - Radiating pain in the shoulder, the arm by its internal aspect, the wrist (in its dorsal and ventral part), and sometimes the elbow. The patient may also present allodynia and hyperalgesia. Pain is felt when flexing the shoulder to 90º and a notable limitation in abduction. Pain increases during abduction combined with external rotation.

- Sensation of frozen shoulder due to restriction of motion; these patients experience pain both at rest and during motion, especially when reaching for overhead objects.
- Possible causes:
  - Postures maintained in internal rotation of the shoulder (as when wearing a sling).
  - Efforts in internal rotation of the shoulder (as in swimming crawl style).
  - Falls where the arm is used to cushion the impact.
  - After dislocation or fracture.
- Differential diagnosis:
  - Shoulder in patients with hemiplegia.
  - Shoulder with limitation of movement due to adhesions.
  - Neurological syndromes such as brachial plexus or thoracic gorge syndromes.
  - Wrist problems.
- Affection of other muscles with similar referred pain: Pectoralis, serratus anterior, diaphragm, latissimus dorsi, infraspinatus, anterior brachialis, common extensor digitorum, extensor ulnaris, extensor digitorum ulnaris, extensor carpi radialis, coracobrachialis, biceps brachii, pronator quadratus.

4.3.12.　Subclavian.

- Origin: First rib and its costochondral junction.
- Insertion: Furrow of the middle third of the clavicle, on its internal surface.
- Actions: Pulls the clavicle downward and forward (helps stabilize it during shoulder movements). Also contributes to shoulder depression.
- Referred pain and PGM:

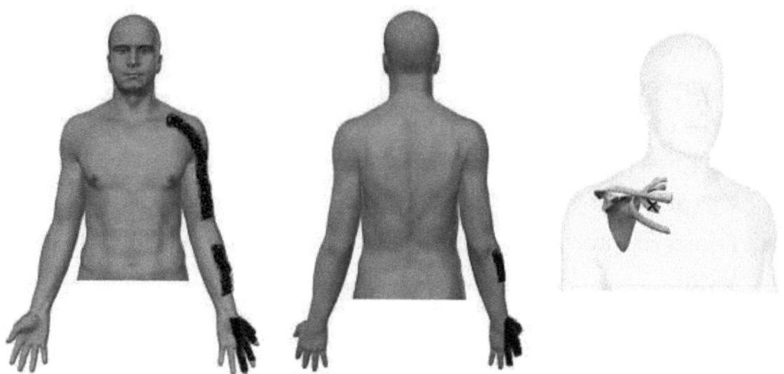

Figure 51. Referred pain represented in black (first and second figure) and PGM represented with black crosses (last figure) of the subclavian muscle.

- Symptoms: Referred pain in the pectoral region, under the clavicle, in the arm (especially in the area of the biceps brachii), in the lateral part of the forearm, and even in the first three fingers of the hand. Occasionally, it may present as a vascular syndrome.
- Possible causes:
  - Fractures and dislocations of the clavicle.
  - Repetitive shoulder movements.
  - Prolonged postures with the shoulder in depression.
- Differential diagnosis:
  - Myocardial infarction (due to radiating pain in the chest and arm).
  - Epicondylalgia.
  - Brachial plexus neuralgia.
- Affection of other muscles with similar referred pain: scalenes, pectoralis major, supraspinatus, infraspinatus, pronator teres, biceps brachii, brachioradialis, index extensor, supinator.

4.3.13.   Biceps brachii.

- Origin: The short fascicle originates from the coracoid process of the scapula, while the long fascicle originates from the glenohumeral joint capsule and the supraglenoid tubercle of the scapula.
- Insertion: It inserts into the tuberosity of the radius and the forearm fascia through the bicipital aponeurosis.
- Actions: The biceps brachii participates in elbow flexion and is a powerful supinator of the forearm. The long portion contributes to the

stabilization of the humeral head in the glenoid fossa and also helps in shoulder flexion.
- Referred pain and PGM:

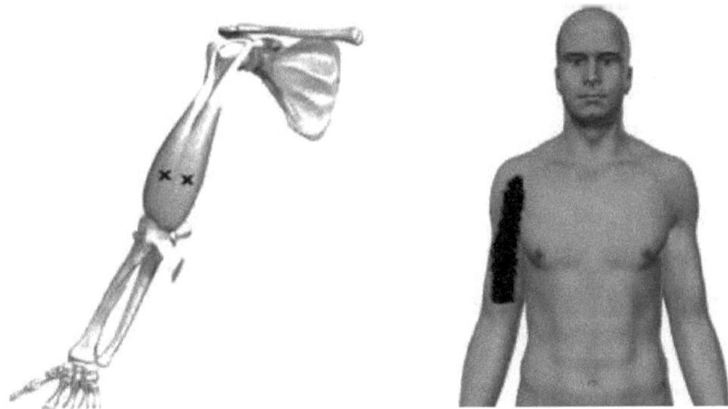

Figure 52. PGM represented with black crosses (first figure) and referred pain represented in black (second figure) of the biceps brachii muscle.

- Symptoms: The pain is localized in the anterior part of the shoulder, being a superficial pain that extends along the ventral part of the arm and up to the elbow flexure area. Movement is restricted due to pain, especially on palpation of the tendon insertions both distally and proximally. Pain does not usually occur at night.
- Possible causes:
  - Repetitive activities such as weight lifting in the gym or continuous use of tools involving prone-supination movements.
  - Subacromial entrapment syndrome.
  - Prolonged immobilization of the arm (e.g., when worn in a sling).
  - Acute overloads, such as sudden heavy lifting.
- Differential diagnosis:
  - Subdeltoid or subacromial bursitis.
  - Arthritis or osteoarthritis.
  - Radiculopathy of C5.
  - Joint dysfunctions.
  - Tendinopathy of the biceps tendon.
- Other muscular alterations with similar referred pain: subscapularis, subclavian, pectoralis, diaphragm, infraspinatus, latissimus dorsi, anterior brachial, coracobrachialis, deltoid and short supinator.

4.3.14.   Triceps brachii.

- Origin:
  - Long portion of the triceps: infraglenoid tuberosity of the scapula.
  - Vastus internus: posterior part of the humerus, over the radial groove.
  - Vastus externus: posterior part of the humerus, from the radial groove to almost the elbow.
- Insertion: The three fascicles unite into a common tendon that inserts into the olecranon and fascia of the forearm.
- Actions: Elbow extension. The long portion also collaborates in the adduction of the shoulder.
- Referred pain and PGM:

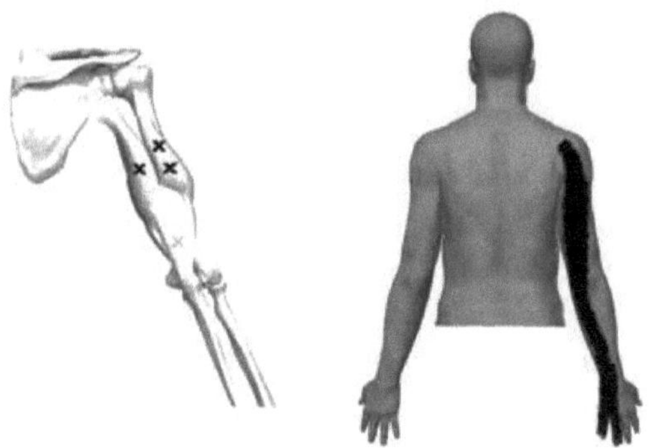

Figure 53. PGM represented with black crosses (first figure) and referred pain represented in black (second figure) of the triceps brachii muscle.

- Symptoms: Diffuse pain in the back of the arm, extending to the shoulder, elbow (posterior and lateral, at the epicondyle) and the last two fingers. It is aggravated by activities that require full extension of the elbow.
- Possible causes:
  - Repetitive movements involving elbow extension, as in sports (tennis, golf).
  - Postures maintained with the elbow flexed, especially without support (driving, playing video games).

- Overloads or prolonged pressure (leaning badly on armrests or using crutches).
- Differential diagnosis:
  - Epicondylalgia.
  - Olecranian bursitis.
  - C7-C8 radiculopathy.
  - Thoracic gorge syndrome.
  - Ulnar or radial nerve entrapment.
- Other muscular alterations: Serratus anterior, angular of the scapula, supraspinatus, teres major, coracobrachialis, anconeus, brachioradialis, among others.

4.3.15. Anterior brachial.

- Origin: Distal half of the diaphysis of the humerus, in the anterior part.
- Insertion: Coronoid process and tuberosity of the ulna.
- Actions: Elbow flexion, regardless of forearm position (supination or pronation).
- Referred pain and PGM:

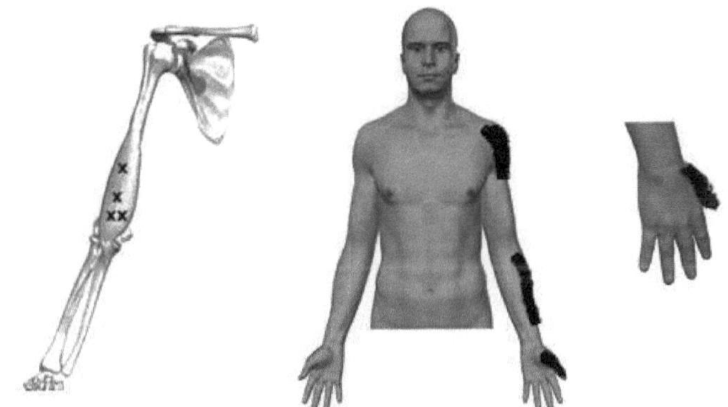

Figure 54. PGM depicted with black crosses (first figure) and referred pain depicted in black (second and third figures) of the anterior brachialis muscle.

- Symptoms: Pain referred mainly to the thumb, but may also appear in the anterior aspect of the shoulder and along the ventral aspect of the arm. Pain does not limit either flexion or extension of the elbow.

- Possible causes: Overuse or repetitive actions involving elbow flexion, such as ironing or carrying heavy bags.
- Differential diagnosis:
  - De Quervain's syndrome.
  - C5-C6 radiculopathy.
  - Rizarthrosis.
  - Carpal tunnel syndrome.
- Other possible muscle alterations include: subscapularis, pectoralis, infraspinatus, coracobrachialis, biceps brachii, brachioradialis, among others.

4.3.16. Coracobrachial.

- Origin: Coracoid process of the scapula.
- Insertion: Medial aspect of the diaphysis of the humerus.
- Actions: Shoulder flexion and adduction.
- Referred pain and PGM:

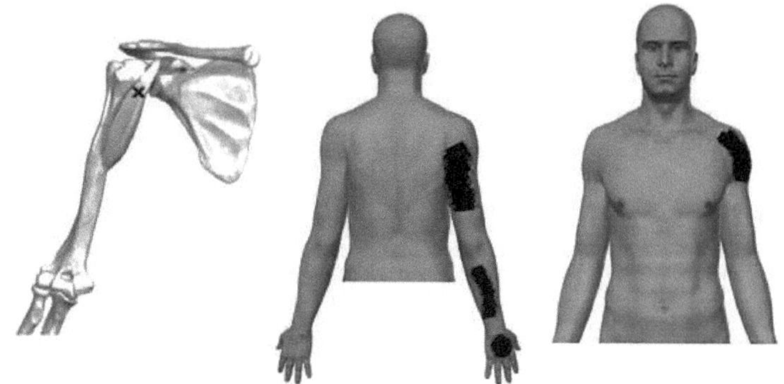

Figure 55. PGM represented with black crosses (first figure) and referred pain represented in black (second and third figures) of the coracobrachial muscle.

- Symptoms: Referred pain in the anterior area of the shoulder, with irradiation towards the dorsal area of the arm and forearm, reaching the back of the hand. The pain does not affect the elbow or wrist, but intensifies when the arm is brought back with the elbow bent.
- Possible causes:
  - Repetitive activities involving shoulder flexion and approximation (e.g., cleaning glass).

- Prolonged postures with the shoulder in flexion or adduction (such as poor sleeping postures).
- Differential diagnosis:
  - Radiculopathy C5-C6, C6-C7.
  - Carpal tunnel syndrome.
  - Brachial plexus entrapment.
  - Subacromial or subdeltoid bursitis.
  - Joint dysfunction.
- Other possible muscle alterations: subscapularis, pectorals, diaphragm, infraspinatus, latissimus dorsi, anterior brachialis, biceps brachii, triceps brachii, deltoid, among others.

4.4. Musculature of the forearm and hand.

4.4.1. Anconeo.

- Origin: Epicondyle of the humerus.
- Insertion: Ulnar olecranon.
- Actions: Elbow extension.
- Referred pain and PGM:

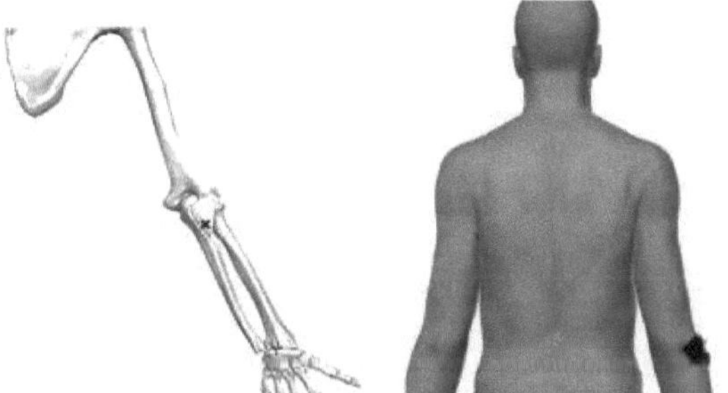

Figure 56. PGM depicted with black crosses (first figure) and referred pain depicted in black (second figure) of the anconeus muscle.

- Symptoms: Referred pain located in the epicondyle of the elbow.
- Possible causes:
  - Repetitive activities involving elbow extension (as in racquet sports such as tennis or golf).
  - Postures maintained with the elbow in flexion, especially if it is not supported (such as when driving, playing video games, etc.).
  - Prolonged pressure or overload (such as being poorly supported on the armrest or using crutches).

- Differential diagnosis:
  - Epicondylalgia.
  - Olecranian bursitis.
  - Radiculopathy of C6.
  - Radial entrapment.
- Alteration of other muscles with similar referred pain: triceps brachii, brachioradialis, common extensor digitorum, extensor radialis longus, supraspinatus, supinator brevis.

4.4.2. Square pronator.

- Origin: Distal quarter of the anterior aspect of the ulna.
- Insertion: Diaphysis of the radius, in its frontal face.
- Actions: Prone the forearm.
- Referred pain and PGM:

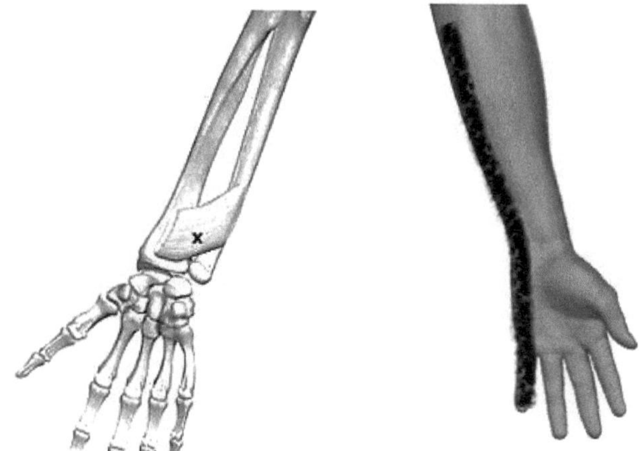

Figure 57. PGM depicted with black crosses (first figure) and referred pain depicted in black (second figure) of the pronator quadratus muscle.

- Symptoms: Radiating pain in the medial part of the forearm, extending to the epitrochlea of the humerus in the proximal region and to the phalanx of the fifth metacarpal in the distal region. Difficulty in supination.
- Possible causes: Repetitive pronation and supination movements of the forearm (such as frequent use of a screwdriver).

- Differential diagnosis
  - Epitroclealgia.
  - Ulnar nerve compression.
  - Joint dysfunction.
- Alteration of other muscles with similar radiating pain: subscapularis, pectoralis, serratus anterior, serratus posterior, triceps, flexor carpi ulnaris, common flexor digitorum, interossei, little finger abductor.

4.4.3. Round pronator.

- Origin: Medial epicondyle of the humerus and coronoid process of the ulna.
- Insertion: Diaphysis of the radius, in its middle portion and lateral face.
- Actions: Pronates the forearm and contributes to elbow flexion.
- Referred pain and PGM:

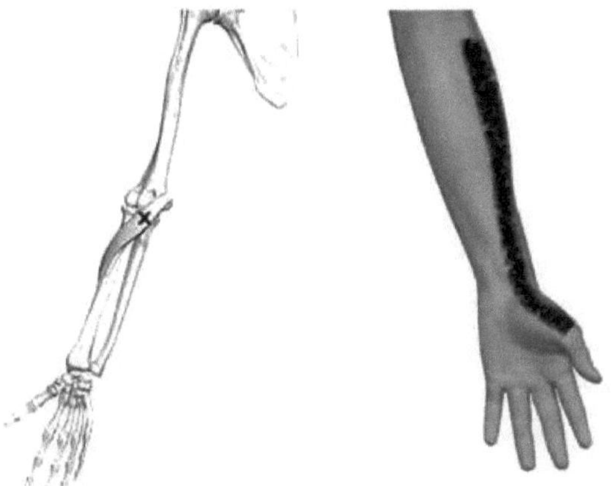

Figure 58. PGM represented with black crosses (first figure) and referred pain represented in black (second figure) of the pronator teres muscle.

- Symptoms: radiating pain in the wrist, both ventral and lateral, as well as in the lateral part of the forearm. Difficulty in supinating the forearm and forming a bowl with the hand, accompanied by a slight extension of the wrist.
- Possible causes:
  - Repetitive pronation and supination movements of the forearm (such as using a screwdriver).

- Trauma or direct compression (such as resting a purse or shopping bags on the area).
  - Locking of the radial head.
- Differential diagnosis:
  - De Quervain's syndrome.
  - Carpal tunnel syndrome.
  - Rizarthrosis.
  - Arthritis.
  - Joint dysfunction.
- Alteration of other muscles with similar radiating pain: scalenes, subclavian, radial carpal flexor, thumb adductor, thumb opponens.

4.4.4. Long palmar.

- Origin: Epitrochlea of the humerus.
- Insertion:
  - Palmar aponeurosis.
  - Flexor retinaculum.
- Shares:
  - Wrist flexion.
  - Tightens the palmar aponeurosis.
- Referred pain and PGM:
  - Pain referred to the palm of the hand.
  - Stinging and/or itching sensation in the palm.
  - Difficulty working with tools due to palm sensitivity.

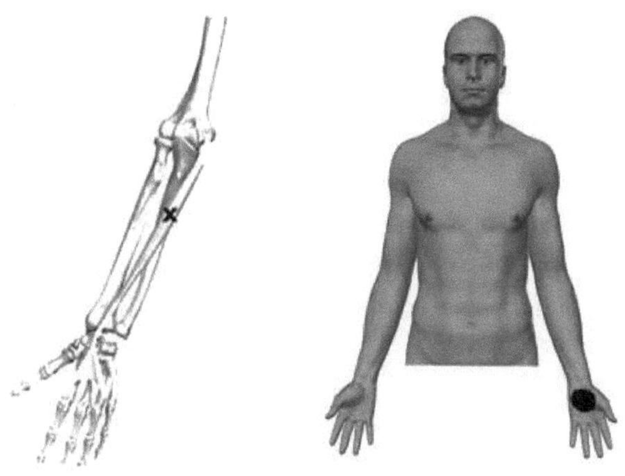

Figure 59. PGM depicted with black crosses (first figure) and referred pain depicted in black (second figure) of the palmaris longus muscle.

- Symptoms:
    - Pain In the palm of the hand.
    - Stinging or itching sensation in the palm.
    - Difficulty in performing activities involving grasping and support of tools.
- Possible causes:
    - Falls with hand support in extension.
    - Activities with the use of tools that put pressure on the palm (gardener, mechanic, tennis, etc.).
    - Dupuytren's syndrome.
- Differential diagnosis:
    - Dupuytren's syndrome.
    - Carpal tunnel syndrome.
    - Sympathetic Reflex Sympathetic Dystrophy or Sudeck's Syndrome.
    - Pain of neurological origin (C7-C8).
- Alteration of other musculature with similar referred pain:
    - Common flexor of the fingers
    - Interosseous

4.4.5. Ulnar flexor.

- Origin:
    - Humeral portion: Epitrochlea of the humerus.
    - Ulnar portion: Olecranon of the ulna and its posterior border.
- Insertion:
    - Pisiform bone.
    - Hooked bone.
    - 5th metacarpal.
- Shares:
    - Wrist flexion.
    - Cubital inclination of the wrist.
    - Helps in elbow flexion.
- Referred pain and PGM:

- They generate pain in the ventral part of the wrist.
- Pain in the hypothenar eminence.

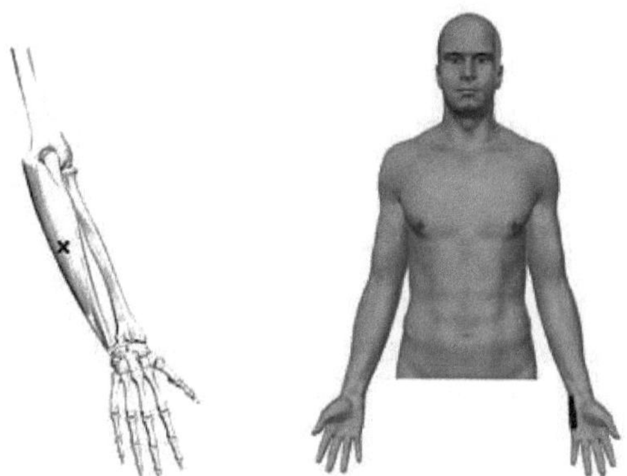

PGM represented with black crosses (first figure) and referred pain represented in black (second figure) of the flexor ulnaris muscle.

- Symptoms:
  - Referred pain in the ventral part of the wrist.
  - Pain in the hypothenar eminence.
- Possible causes:
  - Activities involving strong hand grip (such as driving for a long time).
  - Repetitive wrist flexion and extension movements.
  - Direct trauma.
- Differential diagnosis: ulnar nerve entrapment, joint dysfunction, carpal tunnel syndrome, osteoarthritis, arthritis.
- Alteration of other muscles with similar referred pain: radial carpal flexor and pronator quadratus.

4.4.6. Radial flexor of the carpus.

- Origin: Medial epicondyle of the humerus.
- Insertion: Base of the second and third metacarpal.
- Actions: Flexion and radial deviation of the wrist. Contributes to elbow flexion and forearm pronation.
- Referred pain and PGM:

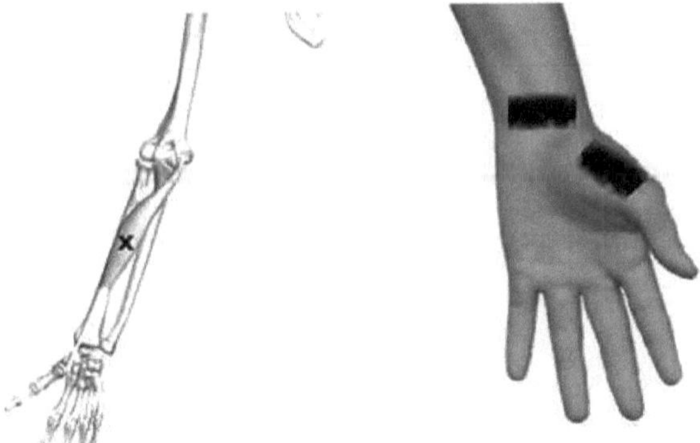

Figure 61. PGM represented with black crosses (first figure) and referred pain represented in black (second figure) radial carpal flexor.

- Symptoms: radiating pain in the region of the tenar eminence and in the ventral part of the wrist.
- Possible causes:
  - Activities involving heavy hand pressure (such as driving for prolonged periods).
  - Repetitive wrist flexion and extension movements.
  - Direct trauma.
- Differential diagnosis:
  - Joint dysfunction.
  - Carpal tunnel syndrome.
  - Arthritis.
  - Arthrosis.
- Alteration of other muscles with similar radiating pain: anterior brachialis, brachioradialis, flexor ulnaris, pronator teres, thumb adductor, thumb opponens.

4.4.7. Common superficial and deep flexor of the fingers.

- Superficial:
  - Origin:
    - Ulnar fascicle: medial epicondyle of the humerus, coronoid process of the ulna.
    - Radial fascicle: anterior part of the diaphysis of the radius, in the oblique line.

- Insertion: On the lateral sides of the middle phalanges of the 2nd through 5th fingers.
- Deep:
  - Origin: Upper three quarters of the ulnar diaphysis and coronoid process.
  - Insertion: Palmar surface of the distal phalanges of the 2nd to 5th fingers.
- Shares:
  - Superficial: Flexes the proximal interphalangeal joints of the 2nd to 5th fingers, and collaborates in the flexion of the metacarpophalangeal joints and the wrist.
  - Deep: Flexes the distal interphalangeal joints of the 2nd to 5th fingers. It also supports flexion of the proximal interphalangeal joints, metacarpophalangeal joints and contributes to wrist flexion.
- Referred pain and PGM:

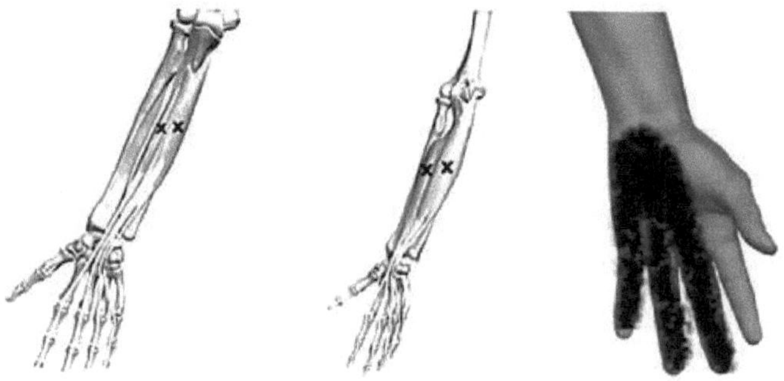

Figure 62. PGM represented with black crosses (first and second figure) and referred pain represented in black (third figure) of the superficial and deep common flexor of the fingers.

- Symptoms: radiating pain in the palm of the hand and in the phalanges of the 3rd to 5th fingers. Difficulty in using tools and scissors.
- Possible causes:
  - Repetitive activities involving hand strength (such as handling tools, playing golf, etc.).
  - Repetitive finger movements (such as playing the piano or guitar).
  - Falls with hand support in extension.
- Differential diagnosis:

- Carpal tunnel syndrome.
- Radiculopathy of the ulnar nerve.
- Arthritis.
- Arthrosis.
- Joint dysfunction.
- Alteration of other muscles with similar radiating pain: pectoralis, serratus anterior, triceps brachii, palmaris longus, interossei, pronator quadratus, little finger abductor.

4.4.8. Brachioradialis

- Origin: Proximal two thirds of the supracondylar crest of the humerus.
- Insertion: Lateral part of the diaphysis of the radius, in its distal portion, near the styloid process.
- Shares
    - Flex the elbow.
    - Participates in the pronation of the forearm, adjusting according to the initial position (prone or supine).
- Referred pain and PGM:

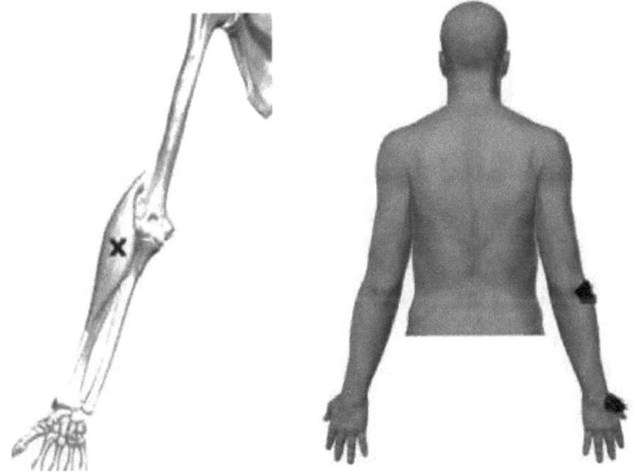

Figure 63. PGM depicted with black crosses (first figure) and referred pain depicted in black (second figure) of the brachioradialis.

- Symptoms
    - Referred pain in the epicondyle and in the dorsal area of the tenar eminence.
    - Weakness of grip, reported by patients.

- Possible causes:
  - Activities that cause forearm overload (sports such as tennis, golf, working with tools).
  - Direct trauma.
  - Prolonged compression (such as carrying a bag on the forearm).
- Differential diagnosis:
  - Epicondylalgia.
  - Rhizarthrosis or arthritis of the thumb.
  - Joint dysfunction in the elbow or thumb.
  - De Quervain's syndrome.
  - Radiculopathy of C6.
- Alterations of other muscles with similar referred pain: scalenes, subclavian, supraspinatus, infraspinatus, anterior brachial, triceps brachii, anconeus, long radial extensor, common extensor of the fingers, radial flexor of the carpus, short supinator, thumb adductor, thumb opponens.

4.4.9. Short radial extensor.

- Origin: Epicondyle of the humerus.
- Insertion: Base of the third metacarpal.
- Shares:
  - Wrist extension.
  - Radial deviation (abduction) of the wrist.
- Referred pain and PGM: They generate referred pain in the dorsum of the hand and the region near the epicondyle.

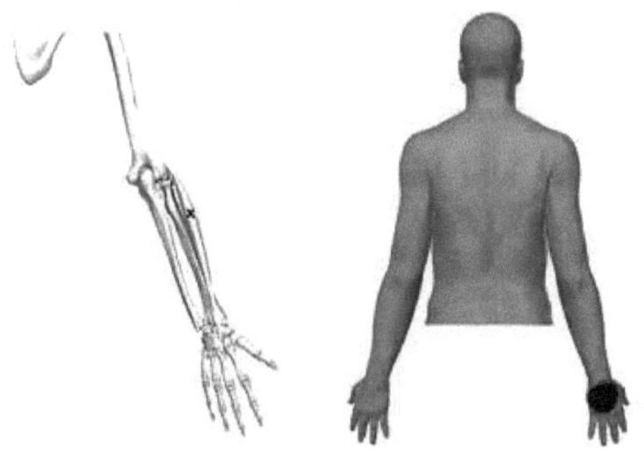

Figure 64. PGM depicted with black crosses (first figure) and referred pain depicted in black (second figure) of the extensor carpi radialis brevis.

Symptoms:
- Weakness of grip with pain.
- Referred pain in the back of the hand.
- Possible causes:
  - Repetitive movements that require gripping force with the hand.
  - Posture maintained in wrist extension, as when holding the handlebars of a bicycle.
  - Direct trauma to the area.
- Differential diagnosis:
  - Joint dysfunction.
  - De Quervain's syndrome.
  - C6-C7 radiculopathy.
  - Carpal tunnel syndrome.
  - Rizarthrosis.
  - Arthritis.
- Muscles with similar referred pain:
  - Coracobrachial.
  - Ulnar extensor of the carpus.
  - Index extender.
  - Interosseous.

4.4.10. Common extensor of the fingers.

- Origin: Epicondyle of the humerus.
- Insertion: It is divided into four tendons that insert in the middle and proximal phalanges of the 2nd to 5th fingers.
- Shares:
  - Extends the metacarpophalangeal joints of the 2nd to 5th fingers.
  - Extends the distal and proximal interphalangeal joints of the 2nd to 5th fingers.
  - Extend the wrist.
- Referred pain and PGM:

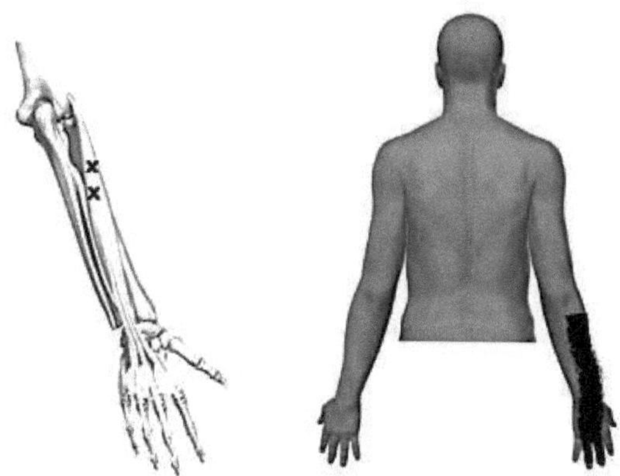

Figure 65. PGM depicted with black crosses (first figure) and referred pain depicted in black (second figure) of the common extensor digitorum.

- They generate pain in the dorsum of the forearm and wrist.
- Pain may radiate to the third and fourth toes.
- Some trigger points also cause pain in the ventral area of the wrist and in the epicondyle.
- Restriction of finger mobility and hypersensitivity in the interphalangeal joints.

- Symptoms:
  - Pain in the dorsum of the forearm and wrist, which may radiate to the third and fourth fingers.
  - Additional pain in the ventral area of the wrist and in the epicondyle in some cases.
  - Restriction in the mobility of the fingers and increased sensitivity in the interphalangeal joints.
- Possible causes:
  - Dupuytren's syndrome.
  - Repetitive hand movements (such as playing guitar or piano).
  - Intense hand-gripping activities (e.g., elastic band work).
- Differential diagnosis:
  - Epicondylalgia.
  - Radiculopathy C6-C7, C7-C8.
  - Arthritis.
  - Joint dysfunction.

- Alteration of other muscles with similar referred pain: Anconee, triceps brachii, brachioradialis, extensor radialis longus, supraspinatus, supinator brevis, subscapularis, pectorals, serratus anterior, coracobrachialis, flexor radialis and interossei.

4.4.11.   Ulnar extensor.

- Origin:
  - Epicondyle of the humerus.
  - Posterior border of the ulna.
- Insertion: Base of the 5th metacarpal.
- Shares:
  - Extend the wrist.
  - Ulnar deviation of the wrist.
- Referred pain and PGM:

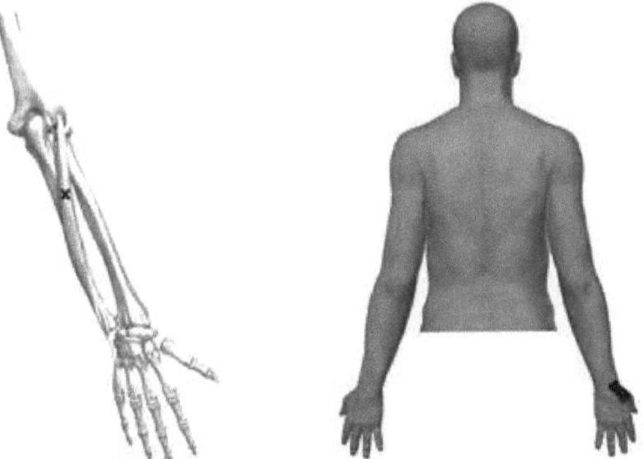

Figure 66. PGM depicted with black crosses (first figure) and referred pain depicted in black (second figure) of the extensor ulnaris.

  - They generate pain in the back of the hand and wrist, especially on the ulnar side.
  - Patients may experience limitation of wrist and hand movements.
- Symptoms:
  - Referred pain in the dorsum of the hand and wrist, mainly on the ulnar side.
  - Limitation of wrist and hand movements.
- Possible causes:
  - Repetitive movements with hand grip and ulnar deviation (such as playing golf).

- Activities that require strong grip.
  - Postures maintained in extension and ulnar deviation (e.g., leaning on an armrest).
- Differential diagnosis:
  - Radiculopathy of C7-C8.
  - Wrist joint dysfunction.
  - Arthritis.
  - Ulnar nerve entrapment.
  - Alteration of other musculature with similar referred pain:
  - Short radial extensor
  - Coracobrachial
  - Index Extender
  - Interosseous

4.4.12.   Supinator.

- Origin: Epicondyle of the humerus and posterior part of the ulnar diaphysis.
- Insertion: Proximal third of the radius, in the tuberosity, oblique line and diaphysis.
- Actions: Supine the forearm.
- Referred pain and PGM:

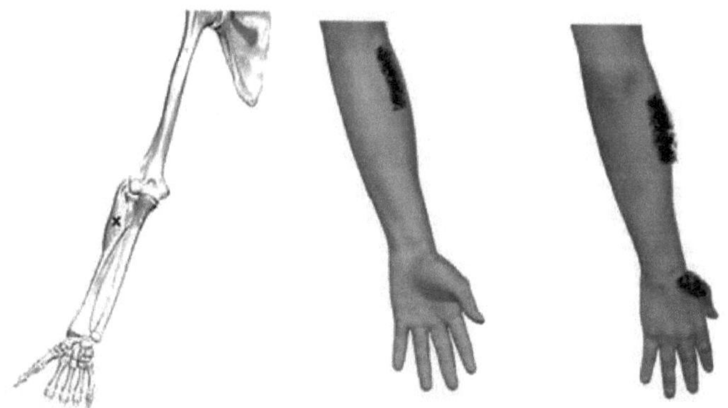

Figure 67. PGM represented with black crosses (first figure) and referred pain represented in black (second and third figures) of the supinator.

- Symptoms: Radiating pain in the elbow flexure and epicondyle, extending to the back of the elbow, as well as in the area of the tenar eminence and the anatomical tobacco cup. Difficulty bearing weight on the hand with the elbow extended, with pain even at rest.
- Possible causes:
  - Repetitive pronation and supination movements of the forearm (such as using a screwdriver or playing tennis).
  - Lifting excessive weights.
  - Trauma (such as when a dog runs off and the owner holds the leash, causing a "tug").
- Differential diagnosis:
  - Epicondylalgia.
  - Rizarthrosis.
  - Arthritis.
  - Joint dysfunction.
  - Radiculopathy of C6.
  - De Quervain's syndrome.
- Alteration of other muscles with similar radiating pain: Anconee, triceps brachii, brachioradialis, common extensor digitorum, extensor radialis longus, supraspinatus, scalenes, subclavian, brachialis anterior, biceps brachii, thumb adductor, thumb opponens.

4.4.13.   Opponent of the thumb.

- Origin: Tubercle of the trapezium bone and flexor retinaculum.
- Insertion: Radial side of the first metacarpal.
- Actions: Flexes the metacarpophalangeal joint, abducts it and rotates it medially, which together allows opposition of the thumb.
- Referred pain and PGM:

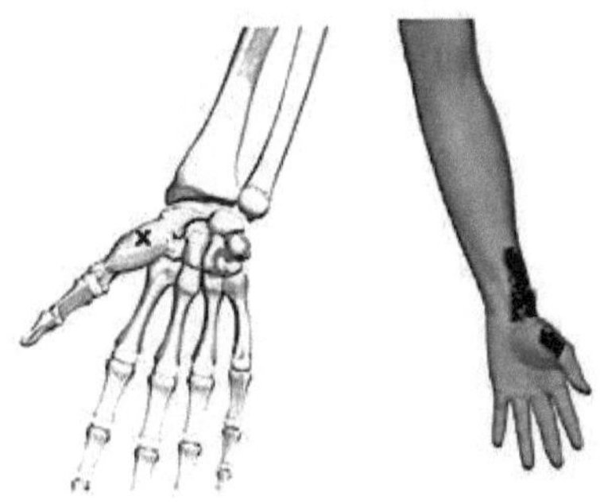

Figure 68. PGM depicted with black crosses (first figure) and referred pain depicted in black (second figure) of the thumb opponent.

- Symptoms:
    - Radiating pain in the radial and ventral area of the wrist and thumb.
    - Difficulty performing tasks involving the use of the thumb, such as typing on a computer, opening jars, holding objects with tweezers or sewing.
    - Patients often report difficulties with fine motor skills.
- Possible causes:
    - Activities that require prolonged use of the clamp (such as pulling weeds or sewing).
    - Fracture or dislocation of the thumb.
- Differential diagnosis:
    - Rizarthrosis.
    - Arthritis.
    - Joint dysfunction.
    - Carpal tunnel syndrome.
    - De Quervain's syndrome.
    - Compression of the median nerve.
- Alteration of other muscles with similar radiating pain: thumb adductor, thumb flexor longus, short supinator, pronator teres, radial carpal flexor, brachioradialis, anterior brachialis, scalenes.

4.4.14. Interosseous of the hand.

- Origin: Each of the dorsal interosseous muscles originates on the sides of the metacarpals between which they are located (one between the first and second metacarpals, one between the second and third metacarpals, one between the third and fourth metacarpals, and the last between the fourth and fifth metacarpals).
- Insertion: They are inserted in the extensor expansions and bases of the proximal phalanges: the first interosseous on the radial side of the second metacarpal, the second on the radial side of the third metacarpal, the third on the ulnar side of the third metacarpal and the fourth on the ulnar side of the fourth metacarpal.
- Actions: They abduct the fingers in relation to an axis located on the third metacarpal. They assist in the flexion of the

metacarpophalangeal joints and in the extension of the interphalangeal joints.
- Referred pain and PGM:

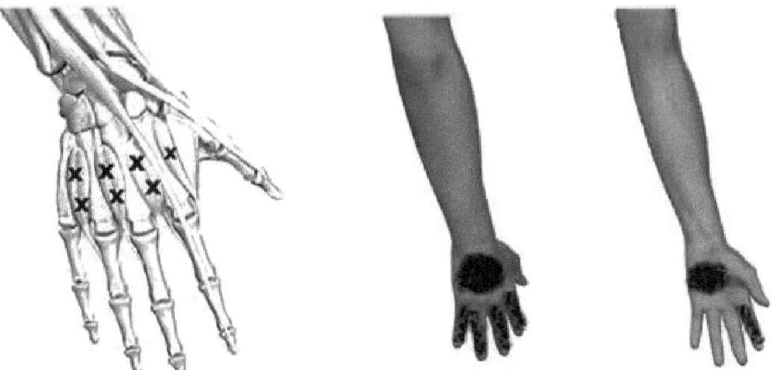

Figure 69. PGM depicted with black crosses (first figure) and referred pain depicted in black (second figure) of the thumb opponent.

- Symptoms:
    - The first interosseous causes pain in the index finger, in the palm of the hand (especially in the center) and in the back of the hand, even radiating to the little finger.
    - The other interosseous cause referred pain along the finger where they are inserted.
    - Patients experience stiffness or difficulty moving their fingers, affecting everyday activities such as buttoning a button or typing.
    - The referred pain of the dorsal interossei, palmar interossei and lumbricals is practically identical.
- Possible causes:
    - Activities that involve maintaining a manual gripper for long periods of time.
    - Arthritis.
- Differential diagnosis:
    - Joint dysfunction.
    - Arthritis.
    - C7-C8 radiculopathy.
    - Ulnar nerve compression.
- Alteration of other muscles with similar radiating pain: Coracobrachialis, short radial extensor, common extensor digitorum,

ulnar extensor, index extensor, palmaris longus, common flexor digitorum, pronator quadratus, little finger abductor.

5. TREATMENT TECHNIQUES.

PGM release refers to a series of techniques that seek to reduce muscle tension and relieve pain associated with PGMs. These techniques are varied, and different practitioners use different approaches to pain management. This section presents some of the most common techniques, based on new insights into the nature of PGMs (80, 81).

It is critical to differentiate between central PGs and insertional PGs in order to select the appropriate treatment. Central PGs respond better to stretching and direct release techniques, while insertional PGs benefit more from manual therapies and techniques to reduce overload on muscle insertions. In addition, rehabilitation of muscle function is key, especially in patients with chronic pain. It is necessary not only to inactivate the PGMs, but also to reeducate the muscle to regain its strength, coordination and endurance. Tools such as surface EMG can help monitor muscle fatigue and loss of strength, facilitating re-education through quantitative feedback (80, 81).

5.1. Approach to non-invasive techniques.

5.1.1. Spray stretching technique.

The "spray and stretch" technique is an effective therapeutic method for treating muscle pain and trigger points (TP), developed by Hans Kraus in 1952. The following is a summary of the key points about this technique, its applications, benefits and limitations, as well as some important details about the application of the spray and ice rub (77, 81, 82, 83, 84):

- Technique:
  - Spray Application: Uses an ethyl chloride spray (or Fluori-Methane as a safer alternative) which acts as a coolant. It is applied to the skin while gently stretching the affected muscle.
  - Purpose of the Spray: Acts as a "distractor" to reduce pain, facilitating the inactivation of trigger points without the need for precise localization.
  - Stretching: The main therapeutic component that, combined with the spray, helps relieve muscle tension.
- Benefits:

- Acute PG Inactivation: Effective for releasing tight muscles and treating acute PGs.
  - Relief of Referred Pain: May relieve referred pain, as in cases of cardiac ischemia, although it does not treat the underlying cause.
  - Versatility: It works well in children, hemiplegic patients, and can be used in combination with other therapeutic techniques.
  - Mobility Restoration: Helps restore mobility and relieve pain in rehabilitation.
- Limitations:
  - Not for All Patients: Not suitable for patients with hyperuricemia, where pain may recur rapidly.
  - Risks of Ethyl Chloride: Although effective, ethyl chloride has health risks, and Fluoromethane, its alternative, also presents environmental risks.
  - Necessary Precautions: Requires careful techniques to avoid skin damage due to excessive cooling.
- Spray application:
  - Initial Sensitivity: Some patients may experience hypersensitivity to cold; this can be mitigated with appropriate techniques.
  - Warning and Demonstration: It is essential to warn patients about the sensation and demonstrate the effect of the spray before applying it.
- Application Technique:
  - Angle and Distance: Apply the spray at an angle of 30° parallel to the muscle fibers, keeping the bottle 30 cm from the skin at a speed of 10 cm/s.
  - Number of Applications: Do not exceed two or three passes without allowing the skin to overheat to avoid excessive cooling of the underlying muscle.
  - Modifications: Adjust application speed or distance according to patient sensitivity.
- Special Care:
  - Facial Area: Protect eyes and be cautious with patients with respiratory problems.
  - Self-application: May be difficult in areas such as the shoulder girdle and neck; professional assistance is recommended.
  - Ice Rubbing

- Method:
    - Ice Application: Use a thin edge of ice and apply it on the skin in parallel strokes, similar to the spray in speed (10 cm/s). Keep the skin dry to maximize the effect.
    - Neurological effect: It acts through a neurological mechanism that inhibits pain, facilitating muscle relaxation.
- Other Uses:
    - Versatility: In addition to treating PG, the cooling spray can be used for joint sprains, thermal burns, acute myocardial infarction, bee stings and postherpetic neuralgia.
    - Animal Applications: It can be used in animals, such as horses and dogs, under specific care to relieve muscle pain.

The spray and stretch technique is a valuable tool in the treatment of myofascial pain and trigger points. It offers a noninvasive and effective option, although it requires careful management and consideration of associated risks. Its proper application, combined with complementary techniques and patient preparation, can contribute significantly to pain relief and improved mobility.

5.1.2. Stretching and myofascial release.

- Stretching technique (elongation) (85, 86): Gently stretching a muscle with trigger points to increase its range of motion without causing pain. The technique should be slow and controlled to avoid pain and spasm. In controlled studies, stretching combined with the spray-and-stretch technique showed reduction of referred pain and tenderness at trigger points. As precautions we will take into account to avoid fast and forced stretching that may cause pain. Use passive and slow stretching to inactivate trigger points. Incorporating facilitation techniques such as coordinated breathing and reciprocal inhibition can increase the effectiveness of stretching.
- Stretching by direct extension (85, 86): Apply direct manual traction to the affected muscle. Often, traction is preceded by the application of cold to relax the muscle and connective tissues. Cold helps reduce muscle tension and facilitates more effective stretching.
- Percussion and stretching (85, 86): Start with passive stretching of the muscle until resistance is felt. Then, light percussion is applied to the trigger point using a hard rubber mallet or reflex hammer. Percussion

should be performed at a low frequency to avoid pain. This technique can replace the use of intermittent cold.

- Post-stretching procedures (85, 86): After stretching, perform active movements that lengthen and shorten the muscle to restore its normal function. Avoid strenuous activities immediately after treatment. Focus on gentle stretching and flexing exercises, ideally in a heated pool to reduce the risk of additional strain.
- Post-treatment heat (85, 86): Apply moist heat, such as a compress or electric blanket, after treatment to reduce pain and promote muscle relaxation.

5.1.3. Voluntary contraction and muscle release methods

Voluntary contraction methods to release muscle tension focus on the combination of active contraction and relaxation to improve mobility and reduce stiffness. The main techniques are described here, each with its specific approach and application (87, 88, 89, 90):

- Contraction-relaxation: Involves an active contraction of the muscle followed by complete relaxation. Gentle contraction facilitates greater elongation of the muscle during relaxation. Improves mobility by allowing greater elongation and normalizes the length of affected sarcomeres. It reduces the excessive release of acetylcholine that contributes to muscle stiffness. For its application we must perform slow and coordinated movements. It is useful in the inactivation of trigger points and in improving range of motion.
- Postisometric relaxation (PRI): Introduced by Karel Lewit, this technique consists of an isometric contraction of the muscle against a resistance, followed by an elongation during the relaxation phase. It may be more effective when combined with coordinated breathing and eye movements. It facilitates greater elongation and relaxation of the muscle. For its application make sure the patient is relaxed. Avoid pain or active resistance during stretching.
- Reciprocal Inhibition: Takes advantage of the spinal reflex where the contraction of one muscle causes the inhibition of the antagonist muscle, facilitating stretching and release of tension. It facilitates the stretching of trigger points and can be combined with techniques such as spray and stretch. It can also influence spontaneous electrical

activity and mental stress. It can be used to increase stretching or as a complementary technique in the treatment of trigger points.

- Hold-relaxation: Similar to contraction-relaxation, but without active elongation. It involves an isometric contraction followed by relaxation. Allows avoidance of movement during treatment. Often combined with manual techniques such as deep massage or pressure release. It is useful when it is desired to minimize movement during trigger point treatment.

- Muscle energy techniques: They include isometric contraction (no joint movement), isotonic contraction (resisted concentric movement) and isolytic contraction (resisted eccentric movement). They improve joint mobility, stretch tight muscles and balance neuromuscular relationships. Each technique has a specific approach to mobilizing and stretching muscles. These osteopathic techniques are used to address restricted joints and improve overall mobility.

5.1.4. Trigger point pressure release

The term "trigger point pressure release" replaces the old concept of "ischemic compression". This method is effective for treating central trigger points, but its efficacy on insertional trigger points remains to be investigated. Although the trigger point core already suffers from severe hypoxia, and such intense pressure is not needed to cause ischemia, the goal of the treatment is to release the contracted sarcomeres. Formerly known as ischemic compression, this technique was also called "myotherapy" by Prudden, and was adopted by a group of professionals called myotherapists. However, we recommend trigger point pressure release, as it is a less invasive technique than ischemic compression and employs the concept of barrier release. This technique appears to be equally or more clinically effective, with less risk of additional ischemia. It is also less aggressive and allows patients to learn to self-apply the treatment, although it requires greater manual dexterity (87, 88, 89, 90).

To apply pressure release, the clinician stretches the muscle until resistance is felt and then applies gradually increasing gentle pressure over the trigger point until a defined barrier is encountered. At this point, the patient may feel some discomfort, but no pain. Pressure is maintained until the tension under the finger decreases, then pressure is increased to reach a new barrier and the process is repeated. This technique is painless and avoids increasing tension on insertional trigger points. It is especially useful in thin muscles such as the infraspinatus. The effectiveness of this approach can be enhanced with complementary techniques that do not cause pain. For example, maintaining tension on the muscle during the procedure and using alternating contraction-relaxation maneuvers can enhance trigger point release. However, the technique can fail if the trigger point is too sensitive, if the pressure applied is incorrect, if the operator applies too much pressure, or if the patient has factors that perpetuate trigger point irritability. Shiatsu and acupressure are similar techniques to ischemic compression, but are not directly related to trigger points. Although often used to treat similar pain, Shiatsu and acupressure have different philosophies and are applied to different pathologies (87, 88, 89, 90).

5.1.5. Deep rubbing massage and other massage techniques.

Deep rubbing massage, also known as longitudinal massage, was one of the first widely accepted techniques for treating fibrositis, the descriptions of which coincide with myofascial trigger points. This method, widely used in the early 20th century, is effective in inactivating central trigger points when applied manually in a direct manner, without causing excessive joint movement (91, 92, 93, 94).

Deep rubbing massage should be performed by trained clinicians with attention to restrictive barriers. The patient should be in a comfortable position, with the muscle completely relaxed and stretched without pain. If the subcutaneous tissues are tight, lubricant should be applied. The thumbs or one finger of each hand are placed to trap the tight band just beyond the trigger point. Pressure is applied until a restrictive barrier is reached, stretching the shortened sarcomeres and releasing the tension. Massage should be continued along the taut band to the insertion of the muscle to restore its normal length. The next stroke of the massage is performed in the opposite direction, from the other side of the nodule, to release more tension. It is important to avoid excessive pressure or speed, as this may damage the contracting nodes and increase pain. The breakdown of sarcolemma at the contraction nodes may explain the effectiveness of deep massage. Studies have shown that deep massage relieves symptoms in most patients and may cause a transient increase in serum myoglobin levels (91, 92, 93, 94).

Unlike Cyriax deep friction massage, which is applied perpendicular to the muscle fibers, deep rubbing massage relies on stretching shortened sarcomeres. Cyriax is more closely related to strumming, which is applied to central trigger points near the middle of the muscle. Strumming involves sliding the finger across the taut bands, perpendicular to the muscle fibers, until the trigger point nodule is encountered. Light contact is maintained until the tissue is released, and then pulled perpendicularly to release the tension. This technique is useful in muscles such as the masseter and medial pterygoid. Friction massage focuses on mobilizing the superficial tissues over the underlying structures to improve their mobility. Although it is used as a complementary technique, it is not considered a specific therapy for trigger points (91, 92, 93, 94).

Periosteal therapy, applied to bony prominences, involves a rhythmic and disjointed massage technique that should not be confused with myofascial trigger point treatment. Pressure is applied for 2-4 minutes in waves of 4-10 seconds over the periosteum near painful areas. The efficacy of this technique is based on a different mechanism than the pressure points described for myofascial trigger points (91, 92, 93, 94).

5.1.6. Indirect Techniques

- Tension and Counter-tension (Janes'): This osteopathic technique uses body positioning to release hypersensitive points, which are considered foci of constriction in myofascial tissues. Although the points described by Janes may appear different from those in fibromyalgia, they could be related to insertional myofascial PGs. Hypersensitive points are identified in antagonist muscles and are treated by positioning the body in a comfort position that reduces tension on the hypersensitive point. The position is held for approximately 90 seconds until the point is released, and then slowly returned to the neutral position. One could investigate whether Janes hypersensitive points correlate with insertional PGs and compare the efficacy of PG-specific treatment with positional release (91, 92, 93, 94).

- Myofascial Release: This therapeutic system combines principles of soft tissue techniques, muscle energy and inherent craniosacral strength. It uses subjective energy transfer to treat myofascial PGs. Although it is based on promising theoretical principles, more research is needed to evaluate its actual efficacy and whether it provides additional benefits compared with specific treatments for PGMs (91, 92, 93, 94).

5.1.7. Accessory Techniques

- Synchronous breathing: Slow, deep exhalation helps muscle relaxation, while inspiration can facilitate muscle activity. By coordinating breathing with muscle stretching techniques, the contraction phase can be synchronized with inspiration and the relaxation phase with expiration. This can be particularly useful in the relaxation of neck muscles and other areas. Some studies show that PG activity may increase with inspiration and decrease with expiration (95, 96).
- Directed eye movements: The direction of gaze can facilitate movement in the desired direction and inhibit movement in the opposite direction. This can be applied to improve stretching techniques. Looking in the direction of the movement needed to relax a specific muscle can facilitate the release of tension in that muscle. There is a relationship between eye movement frequency and respiratory rate, although more research specific to this phenomenon is needed (95, 96).
- Rolled clamp: This technique is used to relieve panniculosis and can be useful in the diagnosis and treatment of this condition. It is most effective on the shoulders and upper back, and less so in other areas such as the buttocks. The reason behind its effectiveness is not yet completely clear (95, 96).
- Biofeedback: Biofeedback can help patients avoid unnecessary muscle activity and improve muscle coordination. It can be useful for patients to recognize and control excessive muscle tension. It can also be useful in muscle re-education after inactivating PGMs (95, 96).
- Heat and cold: Increases circulation in the skin, contributes to relaxation, but has limited effects on underlying PGMs. Penetrates deeper, causes vasoconstriction and may be useful for neurogenic pain. May reduce irritability in insertional PGMs. Patients may prefer

heat or cold depending on the type of PG and their individual response. Research is needed to compare the efficacy of heat and cold in the treatment of PGMs (76).

- Iontophoresis and sonophoresis (97):
  - Iontophoresis: Uses direct current to move ions through the skin, with a maximum penetration of about 1 cm.
  - Sonophoresis: Uses ultrasound to conduct substances through the dermis.
- Microamperage: Involves the use of low voltage electrical currents. Although promoted by some manufacturers, there are no well-controlled studies demonstrating its efficacy for PGMs. More research is needed to determine its actual usefulness. These ancillary and complementary techniques may offer additional benefits when used in combination with specific treatments for PGMs, and research remains crucial to establish their efficacy and optimal application (97).

5.1.8. Physiotherapeutic techniques for the management of trigger points

- Ultrasound: Ultrasound is a technique used by physical therapists to treat trigger points (TP). It is based on the transmission of vibrational energy at the molecular level, generating heat in the tissues and potentially altering molecular excitability. Although many clinicians consider ultrasound effective, there are no specific controlled studies validating its efficacy. Common techniques include (98):
  - Initial application: Use a power of 0.5 w/cm² with slow and narrow circular movements on the PG.
  - Progressive increase: Start with a power around the pain threshold (1.5 w/cm²) and then reduce it by half, gradually increasing to the pain threshold without exceeding it. This usually reduces the sensitivity and irritability of the PG.
  - Combination with electrical stimulation: Some devices combine ultrasound with electrical stimulation to localize the PG and improve results.
  - The exact mechanism of ultrasound for PG inactivation is not completely clear. It may involve increasing the metabolic rate of PG or inhibition of acetylcholine release. Further studies are required to understand its effectiveness.

- High voltage galvanic stimulation: High voltage galvanic stimulation uses brief, high frequency electrical impulses to stimulate motor nerves and is generally well tolerated. It can be applied directly to treat PG, often after techniques such as stretching or infiltration. Parameters include (97):
  - Interrupted Stimulation: Increase intensity to cause mild muscle contractions.
  - Combined use: Apply tetanizing current before the intermittent current to fatigue the muscle and facilitate relaxation.
- Transcutaneous Electrical Nerve Stimulation (TENS): TENS is a common method for temporary pain relief. It uses low-frequency, low-voltage rectangular waves, acting primarily on sensitive nerves. Although not specifically designed for PG, it can help improve mobility and muscle stretch by providing pain relief (97).
- Pharmacotherapy: Management of myofascial pain may also involve medications (99):
  - Nonsteroidal Anti-Inflammatory Drugs (NSAIDs): Although not effective for central PGs, they may relieve post-treatment or invasive technique-related pain.
  - Local infiltrations: NSAIDs administered directly into the PG can be effective in relieving pain by reducing prostaglandin sensitization.
  - Muscle relaxants: Although muscle relaxants do not directly affect tight PG bands, they may be useful for true muscle spasm associated with other musculoskeletal dysfunctions.
- Sleep Management: Persistent myofascial pain often interferes with sleep. To improve sleep quality in these patients, it is important:
  - Inactivate PGs: Treat the PGs responsible for insomnia.
  - Use of Medications: Antihistamines such as dimenhydrinate or diphenhydramine may be helpful, and melatonin may help regulate the sleep-wake cycle.
- Substances and Habits: Moderate caffeine intake can help, but excess and alcohol can exacerbate PGs. Smoking can increase capillary fragility and aggravate PGs, as well as increase vitamin C needs (6).

These combined approaches can provide comprehensive relief for patients with myofascial pain and PG, although it is critical to tailor treatment to individual needs and patient responses.

5.2. Invasive techniques approach.

5.2.1. Dry needling.

Dry needling can be as effective as local anesthetic infiltration for immediate inactivation of the PG, provided that the release response (REL) indicating that the needle has reached the active loci of the PG is achieved. Generally, dry needling causes more severe and longer lasting post-treatment pain compared to infiltration with local anesthetic. The therapeutic effect seems to be more related to the mechanical disruption performed by the needle, which helps to break the contraction loci of the PG (17, 49, 100, 101).

5.2.2. Infiltration.

5.2.2.1.   Infiltration with local anesthetics.

The infiltration of these areas with anesthetic agents is a technique commonly used to relieve pain and reduce muscle sensitivity. Different types of local anesthetics and other substances that can be used in these procedures are described below, each with their particularities in terms of efficacy, duration of action, possible adverse effects and their suitability according to the type of TMP treated (6, 102, 103, 104, 105, 106).

- Procaine: It is recommended at concentrations of 0.5% in saline. Higher concentrations have not been shown to offer additional advantages, although they may increase toxicity and the risk of adverse effects. It is associated with less systemic toxicity and myotoxicity compared to other local anesthetics.
- Lidocaine: Lidocaine 1% can be successfully used for trigger point infiltration, although its effectiveness compared to procaine has not been thoroughly investigated. It has a longer action compared to procaine.
- Isotonic saline: In some studies, it has been shown to be as effective as local anesthetics for pain relief. It is less irritating than local anesthetics when used for infiltration.
- Corticosteroids: Mainly useful in inserted PGs and in cases where there is a significant inflammatory component. Not recommended for central PGs or motor plate trigger points. Repeated use may lead to adverse effects such as skin and subcutaneous tissue atrophy.

- Botulinum toxin type A: Botulinum toxin type A is effective for the treatment of myofascial PG. It blocks the release of acetylcholine in the motor plates, leading to temporary paralysis of the affected muscle. It can cause temporary muscle weakness in the treated area and requires precise injection to avoid affecting healthy adjacent muscles.

5.2.2.2. Preparation for Infiltration.

Before performing trigger point (TP) infiltration on a patient, it is crucial to consider several factors. The operator must evaluate the patient's position, the use of vitamin E and aspirin, needle selection, and ensure adequate cleaning. It is important to make the infiltration as painless as possible and to assess the need for blocks prior to infiltration. The patient's position should be lying down during the infiltration to avoid fainting and falling. This also facilitates localization of the PGs, since the patient will be more relaxed and comfortable, allowing better visualization of the muscle contraction nodes (6, 102, 103, 104, 105, 106).

A low level of vitamin E can cause excessive bleeding during infiltration, increasing pain and causing bruising. To correct this deficiency, it is recommended to take at least 500 mg of slow-release vitamin C three times a day for three days prior to treatment. In addition, aspirin should be avoided for three days prior to infiltration to reduce the risk of bleeding (6, 102, 103, 104, 105, 106).

For the selection of the needle length it should be sufficient to reach the contraction nodes of the PG. Needle diameter depends on personal preference and technique, with thicker needles (0.7 mm) providing greater tissue sensation and thinner needles (0.4 mm) causing less damage. For superficial muscles, a 0.7 mm and 3.8 cm needle is adequate. In deep muscles or obese patients, a needle of up to 8.9 cm may be necessary. It is essential to clean the skin with an appropriate antiseptic, avoiding areas of possible infection and using sterile solutions. Needles and syringes should be disposable or properly sterilized to ensure an aseptic technique. Many patients fear the pain of needle penetration. This fear may be ingrained from childhood. Cooling spray can be used to reduce skin pain. Apply the spray at a distance of approximately 45 cm for 5-6 seconds before inserting the needle. Use strong stimuli (such as stretching or pinching) on the skin near the point of needle insertion. Other techniques to reduce pain may include rapid needle insertion, stretching the skin to minimize pain perception, and using a skin fold for initial insertion. To avoid preinfiltration blocks, pain should be minimized and neuroplastic changes should be prevented in sensitive patients. Diffuse infiltration of local anesthetic or infiltration of the entire PGM area can be performed. The use of 0.5% procaine can also be used; it is preferred because of its lower myotoxicity and rapid recovery of nerve function (6, 102, 103, 104, 105, 106).

The precision technique for localization of the PGM is performed by palpation of tense bands and firm nodules, and looking for pain on pressure. The method of palpation will be flat, pincer, or deep. Maintain hemostasis to avoid bleeding that may cause post-infiltration pain and ecchymosis by applying finger pressure during and after infiltration to control bleeding. Precision is key to penetrating the PG. Sometimes it feels like resistance to the needle. Use digital pressure next to the needle to stabilize the skin and subcutaneous tissues, avoiding needle breakage. Infiltrate all PGMs in an area if there are several, describing a fan or circle shape (6, 102, 103, 104, 104, 105, 106).

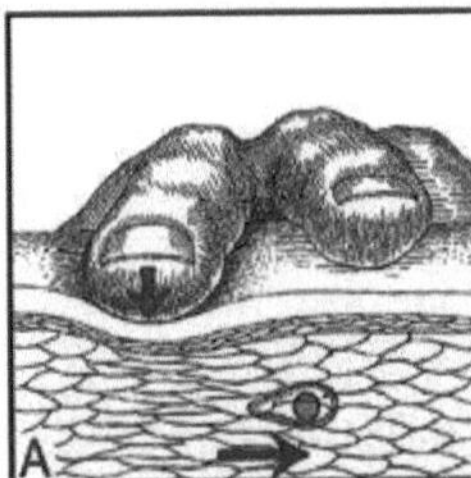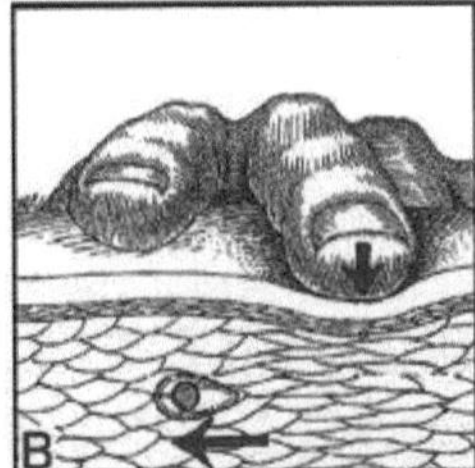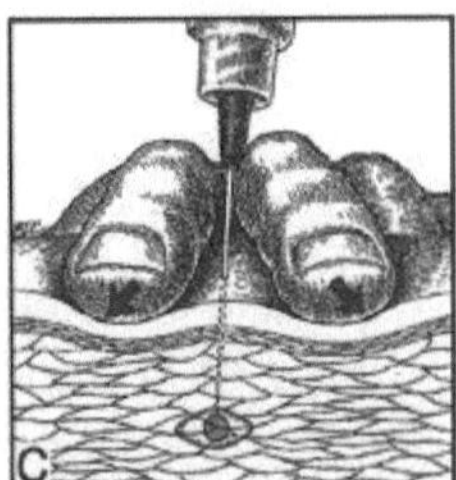

Figure 70. Schematic drawing of the flat palpation technique to locate a trigger point consists of using two fingers to apply alternating pressure to confirm the location of the nodule. The trigger point is then placed between the fingers to prevent it from slipping during puncture (6).

5.2.2.3. Infiltration techniques.

- Hong technique: The Hong technique is used to avoid unwanted movement of the syringe by keeping it firmly in the patient's body. The objective is to infiltrate precisely localized PGs. For the procedure the palpating finger must be held over the taut band to guide the needle. A fine 0.4-mm (27-gauge) needle is used to explore the muscle fibers of the PG with multiple insertions. The needle is moved rapidly in and out. A 2-3 second pause is left between insertions to assess tissue texture and detect local reaction (REL). Local anesthetic should only be injected if there is a REL. This technique avoids damage to muscle fibers and may require significant practice (6, 102, 103, 104, 105, 106).

- Intramuscular stimulation (Gunn): Identification of the PG by local pain and palpation. Insertion of the needle with a dermometer to locate the exact PG. A "gripping" sensation is sought in the PG (6, 102, 103, 104, 105, 106).

5.2.2.4.   Special precautions.

- Contraindications (6, 102, 103, 104, 105, 106):
  - Anticoagulated patients: Except for intercostal muscles with extreme caution.
  - Patients who have taken aspirin in the last 3 days.
  - Smokers: Only after quitting smoking and taking vitamin C.
  - Fear of Needles: Patients with needle phobia should be managed with caution.
- Warnings (6, 102, 103, 104, 105, 106):
  - Direction of the needle: Never direct the needle towards intercostal spaces to avoid complications such as pneumothorax.
  - Needles: Use adequate needles, avoiding blunt needles that may cause bleeding or damage.
  - Needle Insertion: Make sure that the needle does not break; it must be long enough to be handled safely.
- Number of Infiltrations (6, 102, 103, 104, 105, 106):
  - Acute PG: Generally resolved with 1-2 infiltrations, together with exercises to maintain mobility.
  - Chronic PGs: May require multiple infiltrations over months. It is recommended to treat multiple related PGs in the same session if possible.
  - Fibromyalgia: Often requires repeated infiltrations every 6-8 weeks.
  - Ligament sprains: Procaine (0.5% or 1%) is used to relieve pain in ankle and wrist sprains, preferably within the first 12 hours after the trauma. The joint should be moved gently and protected with a brace to avoid pain.

These procedures and recommendations are essential to perform infiltrations safely and effectively, adapting to the individual patient's needs and avoiding complications.

5.2.2.5. Post-infiltration procedures.

After infiltration, the patient should actively move the infiltrated muscles throughout their entire length. This includes full stretches to reach maximal shortening and stretching positions. This stretching should be done slowly to facilitate further release. Subsequent stretching helps normalize the length of the sarcomeres in the affected muscle fibers, relieves tension and can eliminate palpable tight bands. It also teaches the patient how to stretch at home and helps restore normal muscle mobility. Applying cooling spray can help during initial stretching to reduce pain. It should be followed by local thermotherapy (moist heat) to relieve post-infiltration pain (6, 102, 103, 104, 105, 106).

5.2.2.6. Reasons for treatment failure.

- Misdiagnosis and perpetuating factors: ignoring the factors that perpetuate pain is a common cause of treatment failure.
- Incorrect treatment of the pg: infiltrating a latent pg instead of an active one or puncturing near the pg instead of directly into it may result in incomplete relief.
- Use of inadequate needles and solutions: using thin needles or solutions with irritating preservatives may reduce the effectiveness of the treatment.
- Omission of active mobility and home exercises: not performing active movements post-infiltration and omitting passive stretching exercises may compromise treatment results.

5.2.2.7. Corrective actions.

- Identification and resolution of perpetuating factors: it is crucial to identify and address factors that perpetuate myofascial pain.
- Patient education: patients should learn about proper muscle management, stretching and applying moist heat at home. they should also practice good posture and avoid movements that perpetuate the pain.
- Patient compliance: lack of compliance may be due to over-enthusiasm, mistakes in exercise performance, or lack of interest and

motivation. it is essential to educate and motivate the patient, and to monitor and adjust their exercise program as needed.

- Appropriate activities: strenuous activities should be avoided during the period of post-infiltration pain and promote gentle, normal muscle use. patients should also avoid movements that perpetuate pain and learn to perform activities in a manner that does not cause harmful stress.

This comprehensive approach focuses not only on immediate treatment of PG, but also on ongoing patient education and modification of behaviors that may be contributing to their chronic pain.

5.2.3. Therapeutic exercises.

Exercises aimed at treating myofascial trigger points (MTrPs) focus on lengthening, strengthening and conditioning specific muscles. The key to relieving myofascial pain is stretching the affected muscles, as it improves muscle condition and endurance, decreasing the risk of developing MTrPs. However, in patients with active PGMs, strengthening or conditioning exercises may exacerbate symptoms (39, 44, 108, 109).

The choice of exercise depends on the irritability of the PGMs. If there is pain at rest, gentle activities, such as rhythmic stretching in warm water, are recommended. As the PGMs become inactivated, strengthening exercises can be progressed gradually, starting with eccentric contractions, which generate greater force with less energy expenditure than concentric contractions. It is essential that the exercises be considered as a "prescription", specifying type, dosage, repetitions and frequency. Stretching should be performed daily, and if any exercise increases pain, it should be reduced or interrupted. Muscle strengthening includes isometric or isotonic contractions, with isotonic movement being preferable. Eccentric contractions, by lengthening the muscle under controlled load, are recommended to avoid overloading. Conditioning exercises, such as swimming or cycling, are useful to maintain physical fitness and avoid reactivation of PGMs (39, 44, 108, 109).

Throughout this book we have explored in depth the complex and multifaceted topic of myofascial trigger points, from their definition and pathophysiology to the most advanced methods of diagnosis and treatment. These trigger points represent a common but often underdiagnosed cause of musculoskeletal pain, affecting the quality of life of millions of people worldwide. Understanding their origin, evolution and treatment is crucial for the development of effective therapeutic strategies. Trigger point treatment should be comprehensive, ranging from manual therapies, therapeutic exercises and dry needling or infiltration techniques, to patient education and management of psychological and emotional factors that may influence pain. The combination of these multidimensional strategies not only provides symptomatic relief, but also seeks to address the underlying causes to prevent recurrences. In addition, it is important to recognize that the field of myofascial pain and trigger points continues to evolve. Scientific research continues to expand our knowledge, offering new insights and refining existing techniques. In this regard, the future of trigger point treatment is shaping up to be more personalized care, using advanced technologies for diagnosis and therapeutic approaches that are more precise and effective.

In summary, the management of myofascial trigger points requires an interdisciplinary and evidence-based approach, in which healthcare professionals play a key role. This book has been an effort to provide the tools and knowledge necessary to meet this clinical challenge with confidence and competence, with the ultimate goal of improving the quality of life of those with myofascial pain. Understanding and effectively treating trigger points will not only alleviate pain, but also restore functionality and overall well-being for patients. In the future, research and clinical practice will continue to contribute to refining therapeutic strategies, thus ensuring that myofascial trigger points are treated optimally and efficiently.

BIBLIOGRAPHIC REFERENCES.

1. Gallego, T. (2007). Theoretical bases and fundamentals of physical therapy. Panamericana. ISBN: 978-84-7903-976-9
2. Meliá, J.F. (2008). History of physiotherapy. ISBN: 978-84-612-2984-0
3. Raposo, I., et al. (2001). Physiotherapy in Spain during the nineteenth and twentieth centuries until the integration into university schools of physiotherapy. 23(4): 206-217.
4. Chillón, R., Rebollo, J., Meroño, A.J. (2008). Approach to the history of Spanish physiotherapy from documentary sources. Revista cuestiones de fisioterapia. 37(3).
5. Ministry of Health and Consumption (2002). Real decreto 1001/2002, de 27 de septiembre, por el que se aprueban los estatutos generales del consejo general de colegios de fisioterapeutas. Madrid.
6. Simons, D.G., Travell, J.G., Simons, L.S. (2002). Myofascial pain and dysfunction: The trigger point manual. Upper half of the body, 2ed. Madrid: Editorial Médica Panamericana. ISBN: 9788479035754.
7. Simons D.G. (2004). New aspects of myofascial trigger points: etiological and clinical. J Musculoskelet Pain. 12(3-4): 15-21.
8. Iturriga, V., Bornhardt, T., Hermosilla, L. and Avila, M. (2014). Prevalence of Myofascial Pain in Masticatory and Cervical Muscles in a Center Specializing in Temporomandibular Disorders and Orofacial Pain. Int. J. Odontostomat, 8(3), 413-417.
9. Muñoz, J.P., Alpizar, E. (2016). Myofascial syndrome. Medicina legal de Costa Rica. 33(1).
10. Fleckenstein, J., Zaps, D., Ruger, L.J., Lehmeyer, L., Freiberg, F., Lang, P.M., etal. (2010). Discrepancy between prevalence and perceived effectiveness of treatment methods in myofascial pain syndrome: results of a cross-sectional, nationwide survey. BMC Musculoskelet Disord. 11: 11-32.
11. Chien, J. J., Bajwa, Z. H. (2008). What is mechanical back pain and how best to treat it? Current Pain and Headache Reports, 12(5): 406-411.
12. Fernández, C., Alonso, C., Miangolarra, J.C. (2007). Myofascial trigger points in subjects presenting with mechanical neck pain: A blinded, controlled study. Manual Therapy. 12(1): 29-33.
13. Sanita, P., De Alentar, F. (2009). Myofascial pain syndrome as a contributing factor in patients with chronic headaches. Journal of Musculoskeletal Pain. 17(1): 15-25.

14. Borg-Stein, J. (2002). Cervical myofascial pain and headache. Current Pain and Headache Reports. 6(4): 324-330.

15. Lucas, K., Rich, P., Polus, B. (2008). How common are latent myofascial trigger points in the scapular positioning muscles? Journal of Musculoskeletal Pain. 16(4): 279 286.

16. Affaitati, G., Costantini, R., Fabrizio, A., et al. (2011). Effects of treatment of peripheral pain generators in fibromyalgia patients. European Journal of Pain, 15(1): 61-69.

17. Mayoral, O., Salvat, I. (2021). Invasive physiotherapy of myofascial pain syndrome. Editorial médica panamericana. ISBN: 978-8491103950.

18. Guyton. A.C., Hall, J.E. (2021). Treatise on medical physiology 14th. Elsevier. ISBN: 9788413820132.

19. Corera, I. (2014). Estimation of motor unit structure based on EMG recordings. Public University of Navarra.

20. Moczydlowski, E.G. (2017). Synaptic transmission and neuromuscular junction. Medical Physiology: 204.

21. Villaseñor, J.C., Escobar, V.H., De la Lanza, L.P., Guizar, B.I. (2013). Myofascial pain syndrome. Epidemiology, pathophysiology, diagnosis and treatment. Revista española médica quirúrgica. 18: 148-157.

22. Chicharro, J., Fernández, A. (2006). Physiology of exercise. Editorial Panamericana.

23. Shah, J.P., Gilliams, E.A. (2008). Uncovering the biochemical milieu of myofascial trigger points using in vivo microdialysis: An application of muscle pain concepts to myofascial pain syndrome. The journal of bodywork and movement therapies. 12(4): 371-384.

24. Martínez, J.M., Pecos, D. (2005). Diagnostic criteria and clinical features of myofascial trigger points. Fisioterapia. 27(2): 65-68.

25. Ruiz, M., Nadador, V., Fernández, J., Hernández, J., Riquelme, I., Benito, G. (2007). Pain of muscular origin: myofascial pain and fibromyalgia. Revista sociedad española del dolor. 1: 36-44.

26. Estevez, E.A. (2001). Myofascial pain. MedUnab. 4(12).

27. Hernández, F.M. (2009). Myofascial syndromes. Clinical Rheumatology. 5(S2): 36-39.

28. Diaz, L. (2014). Myofascial cervicalgia. Clinical medical journal condes. 25(2): 200-208.

29. Niel, S. The concise book of trigger points: Professional and self-help manual (2017). Editorial Paidotribo. ISBN: 9788499106038

30. Hernández, F.M. (2009). Myofascial syndromes. Clinical Rheumatology. 5(S2): 36-39.

31. Simons, D.G. (1999). Diagnostic criteria of myofascial pain caused by trigger points. Journal of Musculoskeletal Pain. 7(1-2):111-20.

32. Hong, C.Z., Kuan, T.S., Chen, J.T., Chen, S.M. (1997). Referred pain elicited by palpation and by needling of myofascial trigger points: acomparison. Arch Phys Med Rehabil. 78(9):957-60.17.

33. Hong C-Z, Chen YN, Twehous DA, Hong DH. Pressure threshold for referred pain by compression on the trigger point andadjacent areas. J Musculoske Pain. 1996;4(3):61-79.

34. Moldofsky, H. (2001). Sleep and pain. Sleep Medicine Reviews. 5: 387-398.

35. Gil, E., Martínez, G.L., Aldaya, C., Rodriguez, M.J. (2007). Myofascial pain syndrome of the pelvic girdle. Revista sociedad española dolor. 5: 358-368.

36. González, I., Varas, A.B., García, S. (2003). Objective evaluation of muscle tissue after treatment of myofascial trigger points: A study of 20 cases. Revista iberoamericana fisioterapia kinesiología. 6(3): 109-123.

37. Araya, F., Rubio, D., Gutiérrez, H., Arias, L., Olguín, C. (2018). Dry needling and changes in muscle activity in subjects with myofascial trigger points: case series. Journal of the Spanish pain society.

38. Delaune (2013). Trigger points: treatment for pain relief. Paidotribo. ISBN: 9788499109015

39. Borg, J., Simons, D. (2002). Myofascial Pain. Focused Review. 83(1): S40-47.

40. Alvarez, D., Rockwell, P. (2002). Trigger Points: Diagnosis and Management. American family physician. 65(4).

41. Yap, E.C. (2007). Myofascial pain-an overview. Annals Academy of Medicine Singapore. 36(1):43-8.

42. Giamberardino, M.A., Affaitati, G., Fabrizio, A., Costantini, R. (2011). Myofascial pain syndromes and their evaluation. Best Practice & Research Clinical Rheumatology. 25: 185-198.

43. Gerwin, R., Dommerholt, J., Shah, J. (2014). An Expansion of Simons' Integrated Hypothesis of Trigger Point Formation. Myosfacial pain syndrome. 8(6): 468-475.

44. Dommerholt, J., Fernandez, C. (2018). Trigger Point Dry Needling: An Evidenced and Clinical-Based Approach. 2nd edition. Elselvier. ISBN: 978-0702074165.

45. Tough, E.A., White, A., Richards, S., Campbell, J. (2007). Variability of criteria used to diagnose myofascial trigger point pain Syndrome-Evidence from a review of the literature. The Clinical Journal of Pain. 23(3): 278-286.

46. Wolfe, F., Clauw, D., Fitzcharles, M., Goldenberg, R., Katz, R., Mease. P., et al. (2010). The American College of Rheumatology preliminary diagnostic criteria for fibromyalgia and measurement of symptom severity. 62(5): 600-610.

47. Ruiz, M., Nadador, V., Fernández, J., Hernández, J., Riquelme, I., Benito, G. (2007). Pain of muscular origin: myofascial pain and fibromyalgia. Spanish Pain Society Journal. 1: 36-44

48. Dommerholt, J., Bron, C., Franssen, J. (2011). Myofascial trigger points: an evidence-informed review. The Journal of Manual & Manipulative Therapy. 14(4): 203-221.

49. Dommerholt, J., Mayoral, O., Gröbli, C. (2006). Trigger Point Dry Needling. The Journal of Manual & Manipulative Therapy. 14(4): 70-87.

50. Sikdar, S., Shah, J.P., Gebreab, T., Yen, R.H., et al. (2009). Novel applications of ultrasound technology to visualize and characterize myofascial trigger points and surrounding soft tissue. Archives of Physical Medicine and Rehabilitation. 90: 829-838.

51. Niraj, G., Collet, B.J., Bone, M. (2011). Ultrasound-guided trigger point injection: first description of changes visible on ultrasound scanning in the muscle containing the trigger point. British journal of anesthesia. 107: 474-475.

52. Rha, D.W., Shin, J.C., Kim, Y.K., Jung, J.H., et al. (2011). Detecting local twitch responses of myofascial trigger points in the lowerback muscles using ultrasonography. Archives of Physical Medicine and Rehabilitation. 90: 1576-1580.

53. Lewis, J., Tehan, P.A. (1999). Blinded pilot study investigating the use of diagnostic ultrasound for detecting active myofascial trigger points. Pain. 79: 39-44.

54. Chen, Q., Bensamoun, S. F., Basford, J. R., Thompson, J. M., An, K. N., Ehman, R. L. (2007). Identification and quantification of myofascial

taut bands with magnetic resonance elastography. Archives of Physical Medicine and Rehabilitation. 88(12): 1658-1661.

55. Feng, S., Zhang, Z., Xu, S., Han, P., Yang, J. (2018). Ultrasonic elastography in the evaluation of myofascial trigger points. BioMed Research International. 1-8.

56. Turo, D., Otto, P., Shah, J. P., Heimur, J., Sikdar, S. (2015). Ultrasonic characterization of the upper trapezius muscle in patients with myofascial pain syndrome using acoustic radiation force impulse imaging and shear wave elastography. Journal of Ultrasound in Medicine. 34(12): 2149-2160.

57. Sikdar, S., Shah, J. P., Gilliams, E. A., Gebreab, T., Gerber, L. H. (2009). Assessment of myofascial trigger points using ultrasound imaging and vibration sonoelastography. Archives of Physical Medicine and Rehabilitation. 90(11): 1829-1838.

58. Turo, D., Cassar, T., Harshbarger, D., Gebreab, T., Otto, P., Shah, J. P., et al. (2013). Ultrasonic characterization of the upper trapezius muscle in patients with chronic neck pain. Ultrasound in Medicine & Biology. 39(12): 2520-2530.

59. Zhou, K., Hong, Y., Huang, Z., Tang, C., Wang, H., Zhou, Q. (2014). Characterization of myofascial trigger points in patients with upper trapezius pain using ultrasound imaging. Journal of Rehabilitation Research and Development. 51(6): 901-910.

60. Shah, J. P., Gilliams, E. A. (2008). Uncovering the biochemical milieu of myofascial trigger points using in vivo microdialysis: An application of muscle pain concepts to myofascial pain syndrome. The Journal of Bodywork and Movement Therapies. 12(4): 371-384.

61. Chen, Q., Basford, J. R., An, K. N. (2011). Ability of magnetic resonance elastography to assess taut bands. Clinical Biomechanics. 26(6): 610-615.

62. Jiang, W., Huang, Z., Yang, H., Wang, H., Zhou, K. (2015). MRI and ultrasound imaging of myofascial trigger points. American Journal of Physical Medicine & Rehabilitation. 94(1): 34-40.

63. Reeves, J.L., Jaeger, B., Graff. S.B. (1986). Reliability of the pressure algometer as a measure of myofascial trigger point sensitivity. Pain, Elsevier. 24(3): 313-321.

64. Fischer, A.A. (1987). Letter to the editor. Pain, Elsevier. 28(3): 411-414.

65. Huang, Q. M., Ma, Y. T., Li, W. (2010). Assessment of myofascial trigger points using infrared thermography: A systematic review. Complementary Therapies in Medicine. 18(3-4): 144-149.

66. Sikdar, S., Shah, J. P., Gebreab, T. (2011). Quantitative assessment of myofascial trigger points from thermographic images using advanced image processing techniques. Journal of Bodywork and Movement Therapies. 15(2): 158-164.

67. Hidalgo, J., Torres, M., Mayoral, O., Sanchez, Z., Prieto, S. (2013). Infrared thermography for the detection of myofascial trigger points in patients with neck pain. Medical Physics. 40(7).

68. Alkhatib, B., Sultan, M. A. (2011). Infrared thermography in the detection of active myofascial trigger points. Journal of Medical Engineering & Technology. 35(6-7): 311-318.

69. Standring, S. (2020). Gray's Anatomy: The Anatomical Basis of Clinical Practice (42nd ed.). Elsevier.

70. Netter, F. H. (2022). Netter's Atlas of Human Anatomy (8th ed.). Elsevier.

71. Putz, R., Pabst, R. (2018). Sobotta Atlas of Human Anatomy (16th ed.). Elsevier.

72. Agur, A. M. R., Dalley, A. F. (2020). Grant's Atlas of Anatomy (15th ed.). Wolters Kluwer.

73. Schünke, M., Schulte, E., Schumacher, U. (2015). Prometheus. Text and Atlas of Anatomy: General and Locomotor Apparatus (3rd ed.). Editorial Médica Panamericana.

74. Waldman, S. (2020). Atlas of Interventional Pain Management (5th edition). Elselvier. ISBN: 978-0323654074.

75. Davies, C., Davies, A., Simons, D. (2013). The Trigger Point Therapy Workbook (3rd edition). New Harbinger Publications. ISBN: 9781608824946

76. Finando, D., Finando, S. (2005). Trigger Point Therapy for Myofascial Pain: The Practice of Informed Touch. Healing Arts Press. ISBN: 1-59477-054-9.

77. Irnich, D., Jones, J.K. (2013). Myofascial Trigger Points: comprehensive diagnosis and treatment. Churchill Livingstone. ISBN: 978-0702043123.

78. Peterson, F., Kendall, E. (2010). Muscles: Testing and Function, with Posture and Pain. ISBN: 978-1451104318.

79. Schleip, R., Findley, T.W., Chaitow, L., & Huijing, P. (2012). Fascial Dysfunction: Manual Therapy Approaches. Handspring Publishing. ISBN: 9781909141940.

80. Travell, J. G., Simons, D. G., & Simons, L. S. (1996). Travell & Simons' Trigger Point Flip Charts: Upper Body and Lower Body Pain Patterns. Lippincott Williams & Wilkins.

81. Simons, D. (2004). Reviewof enigmatic MTrPs as a common cause of enigmatic musculoskeletal pain and dysfunction. Elservier. 14(1): 95-107.

82. Shah, J., Thaker, N., Heimur, J., Aredo, J., Sikdar, S., Gerber, L. (2015). Myofascial Trigger Points Then and Now: A Historical and Scientific Perspective. 7(7): 746-761. PMR.

83. Gerwin, R. (2010). A review of myofascial pain and fibromyalgia-factors that promote their persistence. Acupuncture in Medicine. 28(4): 130-136.

84. Kostopoulos, D., Rizopoulos, K. (2001). Manual Trigger Point Therapy: Techniques for Myofascial Pain. Slack Incorporated. ISBN: 978-1556425424.

85. Johnson, J. (2012). Functional Stretching: A Therapist's Guide to Stretching. Elsevier. ISBN: 978-1450412759

86. Lederman, E. (2013). Therapeutic Stretching: Towards a Functional Approach. Churchill Livingstone. ISBN: 978-0702043185

87. Myers, T. W., & James Earls (2010). Fascial Release for Structural Balance. North Atlantic Books. ISBN: 9781905367184

88. Chaitow, L., & DeLany, J. W. (2008). Clinical Application of Neuromuscular Techniques: Volume 1: The Upper Body (2nd ed.). Elsevier. ISBN: 0-443-06284-6.

89. Salvo, S. G. (2015). Manual of Neuromuscular Therapy. Elsevier. ISBN: 978-0323239714

90. Page, P., Frank, C., & Lardner, R. (2010). Assessment and Treatment of Muscle Imbalance: The Janda Approach. Human Kinetics. ISBN: 9780736074001.

91. Rattray, F., & Ludwig, L. (2000). Deep Tissue Massage: A Visual Guide to Techniques. North Atlantic Books. ISBN: 9781556433870

92. Rattray, F., Ludwig, L. Clinical massage therapy understanding. Assessing and Treating Over 70 Conditions. McGraw-Hill. ISBN: 0-9698177-1-1

93. Salvo, S. G. (2015). Massage Therapy: Principles and Practice (5th ed.). Elsevier. ISBN: 978-0323239714

94. Hendrickson, T., & Barker, D. (2009). Deep Tissue Massage Treatment: A Handbook for Massage Therapists. Lippincott Williams & Wilkins. ISBN: 978 0781795746.

95. Chaitow, L. (2010). Modern Neuromuscular Techniques (3rd ed.). Churchill Livingstone. ISBN: 9780702050954

96. Chaitow, L., & DeLany, J. (2011). Clinical Application of Neuromuscular Techniques: Volume 2: The Lower Body (2nd ed.). Elsevier. ISBN: 978-0-443-06815-7.

97. Robertson, V., Ward, A., Low, J., Reed, A. (2006). Electrotherapy Explained: Principles and Practice (4th ed.). Butterworth-Heinemann. ISBN: 978-0750688437.

98. Watson, T. (2008). Therapeutic Ultrasound in Physical Therapy. Elsevier.

99. Galasso, A., Urits, I., An, D., Nguyen, D., Borchart, M., Yazdi, C., et al. (2020). A Comprehensive Review of the Treatment and Management of Myofascial Pain Syndrome. Springer. 24(43).

100. García, G., Tormos, L., Vilanova, P., Morales, R., Pérez, A., Segura, E. (2011). Effectiveness of dry needling of a myofascial trigger point versus elbow manipulation on pain and maximal hand grip strength. Elsevier. 33(6): 248 - 255.

101. García, M., Climent, J. M., Marimón, V., Garrido, A. M., Pastor, G., López, C. (2006). Comparative study of two myofascial infiltration techniques in trigger points: dry needling and local anesthetic injection. Rehabilitation. 40(4): 188- 192.

102. Cummings, T. M., White, A. R. (2001). Needling therapies in the management of myofascial trigger point pain: A systematic review. Archives of Physical Medicine and Rehabilitation, 82(7): 986-992.

103. García, M., Climent, J. M., Marimón, V., Garrido, A. M., Pastor, G., López, C. (2006). Comparative study of two myofascial infiltration techniques in trigger points: dry needling and local anesthetic injection. Rehabilitation. 40(4): 188- 192.

104. Affaitati, G., Costantini, R., Fabrizio, A., & Lapenna, D. (2011). Effects of Treatment of Myofascial Trigger Points on the Pain of Fibromyalgia. Current Pain and Headache Reports. 15(5): 400-406.

105. Kamanli, A., Kaya, A., Ardicoglu, O., Ozgocmen, S., Zengin, F. O., Bayik, Y. (2005). Comparison of Lidocaine Injection, Botulinum

Toxinum Injection, and Dry Needling to Trigger Points in Myofascial Pain Syndrome. Rheumatology Internationa. 25(2): 130-136.

106. Scott, N. A., Guo, B., Barton, P. M. (2009). Trigger Point Injection for Chronic Non-malignant Musculoskeletal Pain: A Systematic Review. Pain Medicine. 10(1): 54-69.

107. Simons, D. G. (2002). Understanding Effective Treatments of Myofascial Trigger Points. Journal of Bodywork and Movement Therapies. 6(2): 81-88.

108. Simons, D. G. (2002). Understanding Effective Treatments of Myofascial Trigger Points. Journal of Bodywork and Movement Therapies. 6(2): 81-88.

109. Hanten, W. P., Olson, S. L., Butts, N. L., & Nowicki, A. L. (2000). Effectiveness of a Home Program of Ischemic Pressure Followed by Sustained Stretch for Treatment of Myofascial Trigger Points. Physical Therapy. 80(10): 997-1003.

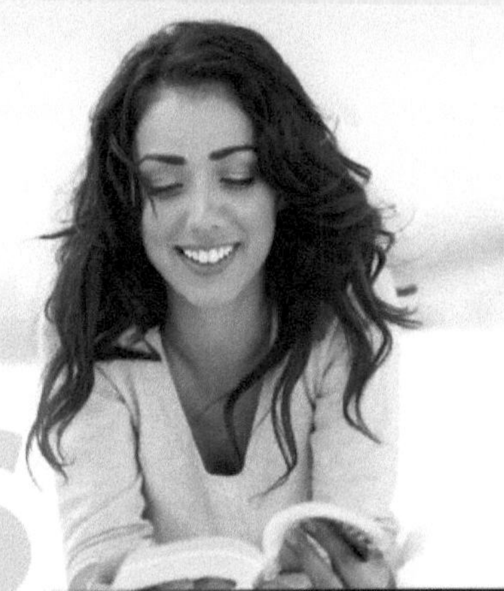

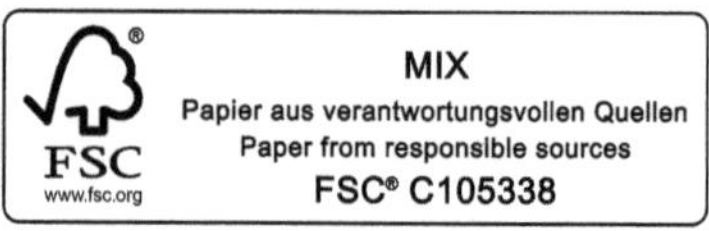

Printed by Books on Demand GmbH, Norderstedt / Germany